Secrets
of Naturally Youthful
Health and Vitality

Samuel Homola, D.C.

Foreword by
Paul-Emile Chevrefils, M.D.

Parker Publishing Company, Inc.
West Nyack, New York

Other books by the author . . .

Bonesetting, Chiropractic, and Cultism
Backache: Home Treatment and Prevention
Muscle Training for Athletes
A Chiropractor's Treasury of Health Secrets

Library of Congress
Catalog Card Number: 70-152523

PRINTED IN THE UNITED STATES OF AMERICA
ISBN–13-797514-7
B&P

A Medical Doctor's Foreword

As a practicing physician, I have always been much concerned with the progressive intoxication of men, women, and children by chemicals and preservatives in foods, unnecessary drugs, impure drinking water, and compulsory treatment with obsolete vaccinations. For this reason, I do appreciate books that offer instructions in how to build good health by observing the laws of nature.

This new book by Samuel Homola outlines a health-building program that will surely help to improve your health and prolong your life. He shows clearly and simply how you can recapture and keep the qualities of youth, how to relieve fatigue and increase your potential for life by caring for your body with natural, everyday living habits.

Secrets of Naturally Youthful Health and Vitality will make a valuable and permanent addition to your bookshelf. You cannot afford to be without it. I sincerely recommend it to everyone who seeks a way to add years to his life without surgical, hospital, or medical intervention.

Paul-Emile Chevrefils, M.D.

11

To Martha with love,

for all her patience and confidence

Acknowledgments

A special thanks to Carole Williams, Pat Turner, Dennis Pledger, Jane Hartzog, Pam Hartzog, Betty Rowell, Jimmy Rowell, Mary Harper, and George Wheeler for posing for the photographs in this book.

All of the line drawings were prepared by Bibiana Neal.

What This Book Can Do for You

When a healthy-looking former athlete dropped dead at an early age, a close friend asked, "What's the use? If good living habits didn't help him, what good will they do me?"

No one can guarantee that you will live to a ripe old age, even if you take the best possible care of yourself. The human body can be born with defects that can result in a fatal "internal accident" at any age. Your chances of living a long life are greatly enhanced, however, if you develop good living habits for youthful health and vitality.

If you do *not* take good physical care of yourself, you will surely grow old prematurely, and you will lose the youthful health and vitality that allow you to live an enjoyable and exciting life. Development of organic disease may cut your allotted life span in half through your negligence.

For every "healthy" person who dies prematurely, there are thousands who "die young" or suffer from ill health simply because they failed to observe the rules of natural, healthful living.

Every page of this book reveals important "health secrets" for youthful living. No matter what your age is, you can benefit from the programs outlined in this book. In addition to the immediate benefits of feeling better, you'll add years to your life and you'll look and act younger. All you have to do is make a few simple changes in the way you live.

Although each chapter of this book covers a different subject, all of the chapters combine to make up a complete and comprehensive step-by-step youth-building program that anyone can follow. Fifteen chapters literally give you fifteen books under one cover. Take a look at the Table of Contents and you'll see the outline of an orderly, progressive program that tells you everything you need to know about how to look and feel more youthful and live a long, enjoyable life.

Every member of your family will be able to make practical use of every suggestion offered in this book. The text is easy to read and easy to understand. Such seemingly complicated subjects as nutrition, the effect of breathing on circulation, controlling the amount of fat in your blood, strengthening your heart muscle, adjusting your spine, reducing your bodyweight, and beautifying your skin, for example, are set out in clear and simple programs.

There is a great deal of *new* material in this book. Chapter 6, for example, presents the new hydrovascular exercises that may be done for special circulatory benefits. In Chapter 10, you'll learn for the first time how to improve your health by aligning your vertebrae with special postures that require you to *relax* your muscles.

I'm sure that you'll find the material in this book so interesting and so effective that you'll want to use it as a *daily* guide in molding your more youthful way of life.

I have personally tried all of the procedures recommended in this book. They have produced favorable results for me and my patients, and I am sure that they will do the same for you by putting more youthful health and vitality in your daily living. You will look and feel younger to a degree you may not previously have thought possible for yourself.

Samuel Homola, D.C.

Table of Contents

*Forget Vitamin D . Vitamin E–the New Youth Vitamin .
Vitamin F–the Heart and Artery Vitamin . Vitamin K Can
Be Destroyed by Drugs . Your Body Framework Is Made of
Protein . You Need Carbohydrate for Energy . Balancing
Fat for Good Body Chemistry . What About Minerals? .
Summary*

*The Biggest Cause of Constipation . A Seven-Point Plan to
Keep Your Bowels Moving . How Constipation Can Cause
Hemorrhoids and Hernia . Forget About Autointoxication .
Foods That Stimulate the Bowels . How to Cultivate
Friendly Bacteria in Your Bowels . Beware of Laxatives! .
How to Take an Enema . Exercise and Sleep . Drink Plenty
of Liquids . Another Warning About Antacids . Pain Means
Danger . Summary*

*Breathing for Better Circulation . Help Your Veins by
Reversing the Pull of Gravity . A Flat Abdomen Is Impor-
tant for Good Circulation . Try Walking! . Using a Rocking
Chair to Help Your Heart . Improving Lymph Flow with
Massage . How to Stimulate Blood Flow with Water . Try a
Sitz Bath for a Sexual Awakening . How to Cleanse Your
Blood with a Liver Pack . The New Hydrovascular Exercises
for a Youthful Body . How to Make "Sea Water" for Your
Tub Bath . For the Robust: a Hot Shower and a Cold
Plunge . Summary*

*How the Aging Process Can Be Checked . "Chest
Breathing" Increases the Circulation of Blood . The Good
and Bad in Abdominal Breathing . Increase Your Lung
Capacity by Stretching Your Chest . Beware of Hyper-
ventilation . How to Breathe Stale Air Out of Your Lungs .
A Warning About Smoking . Summary*

1

How to Be "Young" for 100 Years or Longer

Most of us would like to live for a couple hundred years. Unfortunately, this may never be possible, but there is reason to believe that the human body—properly cared for—could easily last more than 100 years. Biologists, for example, say that all healthy mammals, including man, should live about five times as long as it takes for them to mature. This means that *a man's life span should be about 125 years.*

There are many documented cases of persons who have lived this long or longer. Just about all of us know someone who has lived 100 years. There are thousands of people alive today who are *over* 100 years of age.

From all available evidence, an estimated life span of 100 years is a conservative figure, yet the average man in the United States today lives only about 70 years. Most people begin preparing for death before they reach 50 years of age, and many do not even live that long. Heart disease, cancer, strokes, and other common diseases strike many of us down in the prime of life.

Very few people live to be very old. In fact, *few people actually die of old age.* The individual who dies at 70, for example, has not lived his allotted life span. Chances are he has died of disease rather than old age.

OLD AGE DOES NOT CAUSE DISEASE

Old age itself does not necessarily have to be accompanied by organic disease. Medical scientists now believe that senility as we know it is a disease that causes *premature* aging and death.

There is no longer any doubt that many of the diseases that kill "elderly" persons could be prevented. This means that if the individual begins soon enough to build and maintain good health, he should live to be 100 without suffering from the process of aging. He could live his allotted life span and still be happy, healthy, productive, and full of energy throughout most of his life.

You don't have to be a physical wreck at 40 and then retire at 65 so that you can die at 70. *You can live to be 100 and enjoy every minute of it.*

YOUTHFULNESS KEEPS YOU ALIVE

The "secret" of a long life is, of course, found in living habits that build youthful health and vigor. If you don't take good care of yourself *now,* your body will ultimately break down and fail, long before it should.

"The whole secret of prolonging one's life," wrote Herbert Spencer back in the 19th century, "consists of doing nothing to shorten it." Applied to the way we live today, this means that longevity is simply a matter of replacing bad living habits with good living habits.

Very little is known about the chemistry of the aging process, but we do know that the life of the average person can be prolonged by observing the rules of healthful living. If you smoke, drink alcohol to excess, overeat, and never take exercise, for example, you're inviting the development of disease. And you'll probably live only about half as long as you should.

Unfortunately, it's almost impossible to live a perfect life today. The chemicals in the foods we eat, the pollution in the air we breathe, and the stress of keeping up with a fast-moving society just about eliminate any possibility that the average person can stay in perfect health for very long. But rest assured that if you do make an effort to observe the laws of nature in a program of natural living, *you can live 30 years longer* than you could otherwise.

You can avoid many of the terrible diseases that result in a premature and agonizing death. And you can preserve the qualities of youth long after most people have succumbed to the ravages of age.

YOU DON'T HAVE TO BE "OLD" AT 40

We all know some "old" people who have more strength and vigor than persons half their age. These people are young physiologically—that is, their bodies and their organs still function in a young and efficient manner. Their tissues are firm and healthy, and they have better lungs, better circulation, a stronger heart, and more reserve strength than most younger persons.

It is now well known that the chronological or calendar age of the individual is not a true indication of his health and the number of years remaining in his life. A 50-year-old man or woman, for example, may feel better and have more years ahead than a 30-year-old person who has violated all the rules of natural, healthful living.

If you're under 50 years of age and you're already complaining of fatigue and aches and pains, you're aging prematurely. And if you don't do something about it *now,* a slow but progressive deterioration of your mind and body will lead you straight to a wheel chair or an early grave.

YOU CAN LIVE TO BE 100

If you follow the suggestions outlined in this book, you'll increase your chances of living 100 years or longer. But don't expect to become as old as Methuselah, who the Scriptures say lived 969 years. Even under the most ideal circumstances available on this earth there's a limit to how long a man can live.

Every living thing, depending upon its adaptability to earth's environment, has a different life span. Some insects, for example, live only a few hours after birth. A flea lives about 30 days. An elephant may live more than 200 years. Some crocodiles live as long as 300 years. The redwoods of California are several thousand years old. Very few human beings, however, live longer than 140 years.

Many of the factors that make life possible on this earth also contribute to death. Weather changes and the sun's rays, for example, age the organism by activating its biological clock. And it is fortunate for the human race that this is so. If people lived as long as a crocodile or a redwood tree, the world would be so overpopulated with people that there would not be any room left for trees and animals.

We all want to live as long as we can, however, and each of us is entitled to a good 100 years. So it's important to adopt a way of life that will give you the health and vigor you need to survive. With just a little attention to the way you live, you can be as productive·at 70 as most people are at 40 or 50, and you may even live *longer* than 100 years.

HOW 450 PEOPLE LIVED 100 YEARS AND LONGER

Dr. Grace E. Bird, professor emeritus of the Rhode Island State College for Education, made a study of a group of 450 men and women whose ages varied from 100 to 125 and offered these observations:

"Life for some may begin at a hundred instead of sixty

. . . . Most members of the group had definite plans for the future, interest in public affairs, strong enthusiasms, hobbies, a sense of humor, good appetite and a strong resistance to disease and injuries. As a group they were mentally healthy with an optimistic outlook. None expressed any fear of death. The chief reasons offered for their longevity were hard work, moderation, regular habits, and freedom from worry."

Twice as many women as men were 100 or more, and only eight persons in the entire group were unmarried. All of them were youthful and optimistic in their actions and aspirations.

Compatible companionship can be an important factor in the health and longevity of some people. Dr. Samuel Hahneman, for example, the founder of homeopathic medicine, was a bitter and poor old man who was resigned to death at 80 years of age. But when he married a young French woman, he once again began to practice medicine. He died a rich, happy man at the age of 88.

The French writer Henri Barbusse wrote of a French peasant who, in 1927, was 140 years of age. The peasant's youngest daughter was only 30 years old, which means that he had become a father at 110!

In 1933, the *New York Times* announced the death of professor Li Chung Yun, who, according to the Chinese government, was 256 years old! He was living with his 24th wife at the time of his death. Professor Li was a vegetarian who made daily use of a herb called Fo-ti-Tieng. He also drank tea made from the root of the ginseng plant.

In 1937, a team of researchers visiting Sukhum, Russia, a Black Sea port and subtropical resort with sulphur baths, discovered 12 people who were from 107 to 138 years of age. All of them were strong and healthy.

While I was preparing this chapter, I read a story in the newspaper about the death of a 120-year-old Indian woman who was buried in Glendale, California, in February of 1970.

There are many cases on record of people living longer

than 100 years in modern times. So there is no reason to doubt that the right combination of good living habits will yield the key to youthful health and longevity.

SEEKING THE RIGHT KEY

Although the average life span has increased because of a reduction in infant mortality, elimination of certain diseases, and better treatment for injuries, the chances of the individual living to be 100 are actually less today than they were 100 years ago. One reason for this, of course, is that people are now being "poisoned" by their food and their environment. Food chemicals and polluted air, for example, harden arteries and clog the lungs. Toxins accumulate in the body to cause cancer, arthritis, heart disease, and other crippling or fatal disorders that strike early in life.

There are, however, many things you can do to prevent the development of disease and to clean out your lungs, arteries, and bowels. And, in the process, you'll build the youthful health and vigor you need to live a long, productive life.

A YOUTH-BUILDING PROGRAM

Every chapter of this book contains health-building instructions that should be a part of every youth-building program. So be sure to read the entire book. Once you have experienced the pleasures and rewards of natural living, you'll want to follow "the natural way" for the rest of your life.

No More Fatigue!

Chapters 2 and 3 will start you off by telling you *how to eliminate the most common causes of fatigue,* so that you'll *feel* young again. Anything that causes chronic fatigue can cause premature aging. So what you learn in the next two chapters will give you a good start in your quest for youthfulness.

In Chapter 4 you'll continue on a simple step-by-step youth-building program that won't involve any more effort than making a few simple changes in your daily living habits.

Superior Nourishment and Good Elimination!

Proper nutrition is probably the most important single step that you can take to prevent premature aging. The right combination of wholesome, natural foods will build strong, enduring tissue cells and give you new energy and new zest for living.

Proper elimination is also important. A few special foods in combination with a few special rules, as presented in Chapter 5, will enable you to get the most out of the foods you eat by keeping your bowels healthy and active.

Improved Circulation!

Since the nutrients absorbed by your intestinal tract must be transported to your tissue cells by circulating blood, there are a few special steps that you should take to make sure that every cell in your body receives a fresh, rich flow of blood. Both your mind and your body can benefit from the self-help measures offered in Chapter 6. *You can actually flush your tissues with blood and wash away the toxins of age.*

Plenty of Oxygen!

Respiration siphons carbon dioxide waste from the circulating blood, and it supplies your blood and your body with life-giving oxygen. If you have faulty breathing habits or hardened arteries, however, you may not be getting enough oxygen—*and lack of adequate oxygen can cause premature aging.* The effortless breathing exercises described in Chapter 7 will literally breathe away poisons and cleanse your body with oxygen.

Iron-Rich Blood!

Before your blood can absorb the oxygen in your lungs, it must contain iron. It may surprise you to learn that the red blood cells of the average person contain 20 to 30 percent less iron than they're capable of holding. This means that you must make a special effort to make sure that your blood cells contain enough iron to keep your tissues well supplied with oxygen. You can do this easily by observing the nutritional guidelines in Chapter 8. *Rich, red blood that's loaded with oxygen and nutrients and freely circulating through your arteries will provide a youth cocktail for every cell in your body.*

An Ageless Heart!

What about your heart? It's the heart muscle that must pump nourishing blood through your tissues. Without the special care it needs to stay youthfully strong and lean, it will not function efficiently. If your arteries become hard and clogged with saturated fat, the heart itself may become starved for blood and oxygen. This won't happen if your youth-building program includes the simple measures outlined in Chapter 9, "How to Make Your Heart Last 100 Youthful Years or Longer."

With proper care, your heart can easily outlast the other organs of your body.

A Youthful, Flexible Spine!

The condition of your spine is also important. As a chiropractor, I've learned that *a youthful, flexible spine conveys many benefits that postpone the aging process.* No matter how young you feel, you can't really *be* young if your spine is stiff and weak. You can loosen your vertebrae, free nerves, and stimulate circulation with simple stretching movements that you can do anywhere. This secret of youthful health and vigor is clearly revealed in Chapter 10.

A Slim, Attractive Body!

If you eat the wholesome, natural foods recommended throughout this book, it's not likely that you'll get fat. But if you're already overweight, or if your body is flabby and out of shape, *there is a simple eat-all-you-want diet and a recreational program, presented in Chapter 11, that will cultivate a slim, attractive body.*

Youthful Skin!

In order to *look* young, you'll have to take good care of your skin. A dry, wrinkled, or sagging skin can make you look twice as old as you really are. Don't let your skin betray you. *Keep your skin smooth, pink, and ageless by following the simple suggestions in Chapter 12.*

Self-Help for Chronic Ailments!

As we grow older, there are certain chronic ailments that cannot always be avoided. And how well you care for them will largely determine how active and productive you'll be in the years to come. *For every chronic ailment the human body is subject to, there is a self-help technique that you can use to prevent pain or disability.* Some of the more common ailments are discussed in Chapter 13.

You can grow old without the suffering and hindrance of a broken-down body.

A Good Night's Sleep!

The last but equally important step you should take in building youthful health and vigor is to make sure that you get a good night's sleep. *You can go to bed relaxed and get up refreshed* if you follow the instructions in Chapter 14, and you'll get all the sleep you need to recuperate and repair your body for each new day.

A SUMMARY TO LIVE BY!

When you've finished reading this book, you'll want to read it again and again as your enthusiasm builds along with your new-found vigor. A summary at the end of each chapter and at the end of this book will quickly refresh your memory when you need a quick review.

If you can learn to use these summaries in forming your daily living habits, based on what you learn in each chapter, you'll have the key *and* the combination that will add many youthful years to your life.

SUMMARY

1. Old age itself does not cause disease. If you can prevent the development of disease by building youthful health and vigor, you should be able to live 100 years or longer.

2. If you follow the youth-building program outlined in the remaining chapters of this book, you can recapture the verve of youth. You can be youthful and active long after most people have retired because of "old age" or disability.

3. Remember that any bad habit that causes chronic fatigue or loss of sleep will speed the aging process.

4. Proper nutrition and improved circulation are very important in preventing premature aging.

5. For any youth-building program to be effective, you'll have to pay special attention to methods of improving elimination, breathing, heart action, and spinal health. And if you want to *look* young, skin care and weight control should also be a part of your program.

2

How to Banish Fatigue to Look and Feel Young

Betty B. was only 33 years old, but she looked 50 and felt even older. "I can no longer keep up with my husband and my children," she complained. "I just don't feel good and I'm tired all the time. Life is just a drag for me."

A medical examination revealed that Betty wasn't suffering from an organic disease—and she didn't need an iron tonic. All she needed was a change in her way of life. Her physical appearance left little doubt that she violated many of the rules of healthful living. She was overweight and haggard from too much eating and too little sleep. Fatigue was wearing out her body, and she was aging prematurely from an accumulation of toxins in her body.

In addition to taking the pleasure out of life, chronic fatigue is a common cause of failure in the business and professional world. Take the case of Charlie D., for example. He had to drag himself out of bed each morning, and he dreaded going to the office. "My legs are so weak," Charlie confessed, "that I can hardly get around. If I sit down for just a little while, I get so sleepy that it's pure torture for me to concentrate on my work. I might as well be a hundred years old."

Needless to say, Charlie was the oldest man in the office in terms of production, and there was little chance of advancement in his job. His employer had already threatened to "retire" him. When he came to me complaining of the aches and pains that normally accompany chronic fatigue, I gave him a check list of the major causes of fatigue and told him to follow it carefully for several weeks. In less than six weeks, he was feeling fine and looking much better. His performance in the office had improved so much that he was once again in line for a promotion.

"Follow those recommendations for another six weeks," I told him, "and you'll follow them for the rest of your life. You'll recapture the drive and vigor you once had."

If you suffer from chronic fatigue, you can help yourself as Charlie D. did; and in doing so, you'll eliminate one cause of premature aging.

FATIGUE AND ILLNESS

Practically every disease or illness the human body is subject to will number fatigue among its symptoms. The type of fatigue we're concerned about in this chapter is the type that lingers day after day in spite of the fact that your doctor has given you a clean bill of health.

Since only about five percent of all persons suffering from everyday fatigue actually have an organic illness, the chances are small that you are tired because you are ill.

Even when you are well and active, you do not normally use more than about one-half of the amount of energy your body can supply. With a few simple changes in your way of life, you can draw upon sources of strength and energy that you never knew you had. Think of what this can mean to you and your family.

Increase Your Resistance Against Disease

Freedom from fatigue will also raise your resistance against disease. An overly "tired" body cannot muster its defenses in combating an army of invading germs. There are, in fact, many diseases that develop only when the body has been weakened by fatigue.

More than 100 years ago, Sir James Paget, a famous English surgeon, told his colleagues, "You will find that fatigue has a larger share in the promotion and transmission of diseases than any other single causal condition you can name."

So there are as many reasons as there are diseases why you should make a special effort to banish fatigue.

Basically, there are two types of fatigue that you must cope with every day of your life; one is physical and the other is mental.

THE DIFFERENCE BETWEEN MENTAL AND PHYSICAL FATIGUE

Everyone suffers from fatigue occasionally. When it follows unaccustomed or prolonged physical exertion, it is a healthy warning signal that the body is approaching the limits of its endurance. Adequate rest is all that's needed to restore strength and energy. When fatigue seems to persist for no apparent reason, however, so that the individual literally drags through the day every day, special measures must be taken to eliminate the causes of the fatigue. The first thing you must do, of course, is to determine whether your fatigue is mental or physical in origin.

If you're tired when you get out of bed each morning, and the fatigue continues unrelieved throughout the day, you may be suffering from mental or nervous fatigue. And no matter how much sleep or rest you get, you'll still be tired. Persons suffering from this type of fatigue frequently complain of headaches, stomach trouble, and other "nervous ailments."

Whenever you experience physical fatigue, however, you'll usually feel rested and energetic after a good night's sleep.

Obviously, nervous fatigue is more serious than physical fatigue, and it's the most difficult to relieve. If allowed to continue for too long, it can actually cause disease by disturbing the function of important glands and organs. According to Dr. Hans Selye, the famous Canadian physician who proved that stress can cause disease by upsetting the body's balance of hormones, nervous fatigue may be more dangerous to life and health than the most potent germs.

What Causes Nervous Fatigue?

Nervous fatigue is caused more by mental and emotional stress than by physical activity. Boredom, unhappiness, resentment, marital problems, job strife, and failure, for example, place a great deal of stress on the nervous system. The individual who carries a gnawing problem around in his head day and night over a long period of time may create a form of tension that has many dangerous effects. Abnormal stimulation of the nervous system may "burn up" important vitamins and minerals. An outpouring of certain hormones may disturb the function of important organs. Nerve centers may be excited to the point of exhaustion. An increase in gastric juices may inflame the stomach. Sleep, digestion, and elimination may be disturbed by runaway nerves, and so on.

Nothing is more disturbing to the body as a whole than emotional distress. And when unrelieved stress stems from a situation that is personally degrading or humiliating, it represents a very serious threat to both mind and body.

What You Can Do About Nervous Fatigue

Whatever the cause of your nervous fatigue might be, you must either eliminate it or adjust to it. You should never allow an emotional storm to continue for very long. If you find yourself in an unfortunate situation that you cannot possibly change, you must protect your health by resigning yourself to it and doing the best you can.

I knew a young man who was sentenced to prison for committing a crime while under the influence of drugs. He took up bodybuilding and the study of physical culture in order to "keep busy." When he was released, he went on to win a major physique title, which won him a role in the movies.

A woman with an unhappy but unbreakable marriage eased the pain of her frustrations by writing articles for "true romance" magazines. She eventually sold a book and became well known as an authoress.

By turning their attention away from their troubles in a constructive manner, these people were able to live with their misfortunes and still accomplish something worthwhile. They avoided the crippling nervous fatigue that could have been caused by constant reflection upon their "bad luck."

The wrong job or an unfulfilled ambition is a common cause of depression and fatigue. Albert B., a postal clerk who had spent a large sum of money trying to discover the cause of his "illness," is a good example of what can happen to a man who is unhappy with his job. "I just cannot get enough sleep," he complained, "and I'm tired from the minute I get up until I go to bed. In fact, I'm completely exhausted when I get home at night. I have a headache when I get up every morning, and a backache every afternoon."

As repeated medical examinations had revealed, there wasn't anything organically wrong with Albert. He simply disliked his job, and he counted the minutes during long hours of sorting countless thousands of letters. He had noticed, however, that on holidays and weekends he seemed to have enough energy to go hunting or fishing. When I asked him if he suffered from headache while on vacation, he replied, "Not that I can remember."

Albert B. cured his fatigue and his illness by changing jobs. He worked longer hours six days a week, but he was finally doing something he enjoyed: working on the sporting goods floor of a large department store.

Try a Hobby

If you aren't able to change jobs simply because you don't like what you're doing, you may have to adopt a hobby or an avocation that will satisfy your constructive or creative desires. If such a "sideline" doesn't develop into a lucrative pastime, it will at least relieve your frustrations. It may also offer hope for the future.

I've known many men over 45 years of age who became "ill" when they finally realized that they may never accomplish all the things they had dreamed of doing. No executive position, no fame and fortune, no hope for the future—just poor health, a paid-up insurance policy, a few cancelled mortgages, and premature old age.

Actually, there is no need for despair. Retirement may allow time for development of new interests. A new job may bring new satisfaction. Pursuit of such hobbies or avocations as writing, music, art, photography, coin collecting, antiques, carpentry, and so on, may open new doors leading to fulfillment if not riches or fame. I know a 65-year-old retired "failure" who has been successful in getting some of his work published. "As long as I keep writing," he said, "I'll never give up hope that I may contribute something worthwhile."

Just being alive and in good health is reason enough to enjoy living. The beauty and the sights and sounds of the world we live in have much to offer the senses. But most people feel a need to be useful, to accomplish something worthwhile. Did you ever notice how much more you can enjoy a good meal, a movie, or an interesting book after you have put in a good day's work? You feel that you've earned the right to relax or entertain yourself, and you know that the day hasn't been wasted.

ARE YOU A VICTIM OF HYPOKINESIA?

You've probably never even heard of "hypokinesia." But if

you suffer from fatigue and weakness, chances are you can include this new word in your list of complaints. The word itself means lack of exercise, and physiologists now say that *lack of exercise is a common cause of fatigue.*

Such simple exercise as walking, swimming, bicycle riding, or badminton—even ping pong—will combat fatigue caused by sluggish body functions. Inactivity allows weakened muscles to become loaded with toxins and waste products. Almost any kind of exercise will pump fresh blood through your muscles and wake up your nervous system. Try to strengthen your muscles so that you'll have *more* than enough strength to perform the work you do each day.

Whatever type of exercise you do, begin lightly and then slowly increase the amount of exercise over a period of several weeks. In this way, you can avoid fatigue caused by overexertion and sore muscles. As you become stronger, you'll have strength and energy to spare, and your workday fatigue will disappear.

NERVOUS TENSION CAUSES MUSCLE TENSION

In practically all forms of nervous tension, many of the muscles of the body—especially around the neck and shoulders—are constantly contracted. This contributes to physical fatigue by permitting the accumulation of lactic acid and other waste products released by the overworked muscle fibers. Unrelieved muscle tension can also cause sore muscles, tension headache, and other symptoms.

In my book *Treasury of Health Secrets* (Parker Publishing Company), I devoted an entire chapter to methods of relieving nervous tension and relaxing tight muscles. Be sure to read it if you feel that your nerves are getting the best of you. In the meantime, lie down several times a day and completely relax. Let your muscles sag in order to prevent a build-up of tension.

ELEVATE YOUR LEGS FOR BETTER CIRCULATION

Whenever possible, elevate your legs when you lie down for a rest break. This will help relieve fatigue by aiding the circulation of blood. We all know that movement of blood through the legs is hindered by the pull of gravity. When you are forced to sit or stand all day, a large amount of blood pools in your legs and in your abdomen. Reversing the effect that gravity has on the body will permit stagnant blood to drain out of the legs and be revitalized by the liver and the lungs. The increased volume of clean, oxygen-rich blood circulating through the arteries will then quickly refresh both mind and body.

A short walk will also improve the circulation of blood and aid in overcoming fatigue caused by inactivity. The contraction of the muscle fibers in the thighs and legs will push venous blood back toward the heart, and an increase in the rate and depth of breathing will aid the body in exchanging carbon dioxide for oxygen.

Chapter 6 describes many unique methods of promoting youthful circulation.

HOW TO BREATHE AWAY FATIGUE

Everyone knows that you have to breathe to stay alive, but few people give much thought to the act of breathing. Actually, how you breathe during the day can have a great deal to do with how you feel at the end of the day.

Suppose you do nothing but sit at a desk all day. There is not much of a need for oxygen, so your respiration may be slow and shallow. Three things happen:

1. Your lungs are only partially aerated, so that stagnant air in remote air sacs blocks the elimination of waste products.

2. The subdued action of the muscles used in breathing fails to aid the heart adequately in circulating blood.

3. Venous congestion occurs because of a slow-down in circulation.

All this adds up to an abnormal accumulation of waste products in the body. Chapter 7 will explain how breathing aids circulation. In the meantime, here are two suggestions that will help you combat fatigue and premature aging caused by shallow respiration and inadequate circulation:

1. Several times during the day, take two deep breaths, first breathing down into your abdomen and then high up into your chest. This will open closed air sacs and fully aerate your lungs.

2. Whenever possible, take a few minutes for a short walk. Then lie down on the floor, put your feet up on a chair, and take as many deep breaths as you need to satisfy your need for oxygen.

Such simple aids to breathing and circulation will do wonders for your general health, and they'll provide the natural tonics you need to give you a little extra energy.

Betty V., a 42-year-old secretary who suffered from fatigue, headache, swollen ankles, and backache from sitting at her typewriter all day, reported that suggestion No. 2 relieved all of her complaints. "My work has improved so much," she said, "that my boss lets me walk to the corner and back every day at ten o'clock and at three o'clock. Then I lie down for about two minutes and take my breathing exercises while my legs are elevated. It makes me feel great every time, and I'm always ready to go back to work."

THE IMPORTANCE OF DIET

Enough cannot be said about the importance of diet in banishing fatigue to look and feel young. Although you frequently hear prominent medical men say that vitamin deficiency is rare these days, surveys by the Department of Agriculture have revealed that about half of the population is not getting all the vitamins and minerals it needs. The reason for this, of course, is that many Americans are simply not eating properly. Supermarkets are loaded with a wide variety of nutritious foods, but selection of an excessive amount of refined and artificial foods leaves little room in the stomach or in the budget for wholesome, natural foods.

A deficiency in almost any vitamin or mineral—especially Vitamin B and iron—can cause fatigue and premature aging. A survey in 1965 indicated that Americans were perhaps most deficient in calcium and Vitamin C.

According to *Food, The Yearbook of Agriculture,* "A body well nourished with calcium and other nutrients can be expected to have . . . a well-functioning nervous system, a high level of vigor and positive health at every age, and a longer period of the prime of life." Doesn't that sound exciting and promising? You'll learn more about how to eat for youthful health and vigor in Chapter 4.

Overeating Can Cause Fatigue

Although it's important that you eat a wide variety of foods to assure a proper balance of protein, carbohydrate, fat, vitamins, and minerals, be careful not to overeat. Overloading the stomach can cause fatigue just as readily as overwork.

When there is too much food in the stomach, diversion of an excessive amount of blood from the brain to the stomach can cause weakness and drowsiness that may least for hours after eating. Impaired digestion may also interfere with absorption of important vitamins and minerals. It would be much better to eat four or five small meals each day than to eat two or three big meals.

The Fat Man's "Big Gut Fatigue"

If you have a big, bulging waistline, you may be suffering from splanchnic neurasthenia, which is also known as "big gut fatigue." The strain of carrying around the excess fat is, by itself, enough to cause fatigue. But there may be other, more serious, effects. Weak, sagging abdominal muscles, for example, may allow oversized abdominal organs to fall down into the lower part of the abdomen. This may interfere with the circulation of blood through the liver and other organs so that they become heavy and congested with blood.

Any interference with the circulation of blood through the abdomen can cause "brain fog" and muscle weakness that may make each day difficult to endure.

If you have a protruding abdomen, cut down on the fats and carbohydrates in your diet and do a few sit-ups each day. Chapter 11 will tell you how to trim down without starving yourself to death.

HOW TO ROCK AWAY YOUR FATIGUE

Rocking in a rocking chair is a good way to relieve fatigue while you rest. The light rhythmical contraction and relaxation of the muscles in a to-and-fro motion stimulates the circulation of blood and aids the muscles in pumping out waste products and replenishing energy stores. Also, a shifting of tension from one muscle to another in a relaxed rocking motion will prevent a build-up of tension in any one muscle group.

You won't get nearly as fatigued from rocking as from sitting still. So why not get yourself a good rocking chair? Elderly persons, especially, should use a rocking chair rather than a straight chair when they want to "sit for a spell." Many people, including executives and presidents, find that they can think better in a rocking chair and that they're less likely to fall asleep while reading.

BEWARE OF PEP PILLS!

Physical fatigue is a warning to slow down. Don't defy this warning by taking pep pills. Such pills will eliminate some of the symptoms of fatigue, but the body and the heart will get tired just the same. And when the effects of the pill wear off, you may experience a sudden letdown with overpowering fatigue and depression. You may also become so nervous and restless that you cannot sleep at night in spite of extreme fatigue.

If you take even one pep pill, you may be tempted to take a second pill the next day in order to renew your energy. Then, if you have trouble sleeping at night, you might even be tempted to take a sleeping pill. Needless to say, such use of pills can be very dangerous, even fatal.

Tranquilizers Are Also Dangerous

Tranquilizers should not be taken by normal, healthy persons. Everyone must learn to cope with stress. Most of us have what it takes to get along in this world. The person who takes a tranquilizing drug every time he experiences nervous stress in meeting the responsibilities of life is digging an escape route that may bury him alive.

Stress is a fact of life. It should, of course, be minimized by good living habits, but you must learn to cope with the day's events by meeting them head-on. Look upon every problem or task as a challenge that will lead to satisfying achievement. Don't take the fruitless easy way out by drugging your mind and your nerves. If your doctor prescribes tranquilizers for a special reason, don't take them any longer than necessary.

FATIGUE CAN BECOME A HABIT

Believe it or not, fatigue can become a bad habit. We've all known people who are constantly complaining about how tired they are. Many of them are tired only because of the negative influence of their state of mind. When they constantly tell themselves and others that they are tired, their nervous system sends fatigue signals to muscles, nerves, organs, and glands so that they actually *do* become tired. Even the respiration and heart rate can be affected, so that the individual is constantly sighing and showing signs of anxiety.

Your state of mind has a tremendous influence on your body. This is why psychologists are always telling people to *think positively*. Chances are that the individual who keeps telling himself how happy he is and how good he feels *will* feel good. In fact, the power of the mind is so great that many diseases have been cured by repeating such phrases as "Every day in every way I'm getting better and better." Many books have been written about the power of positive thinking.

If you have been suffering from fatigue for a long time and you take measures to correct it, don't continue to suffer from mind-induced fatigue by habitually repeating that old "I'm so tired" line.

Keep telling yourself that you're full of energy. Get up and go about your chores with enthusiasm. If your fatigue is psychological, it will give way to a smile or a pleasant thought.

OVERCOMING FALSE FATIGUE

There will be many times when you'll experience a false fatigue that will disappear with a little exercise. When you feel "too tired" to rake the yard or go to the gym, for example, you may find that if you give yourself a little push you'll have more energy than you thought. The reason for this is that when the body is sluggish from inactivity, a slow-down in circulation leaves the muscles cold and lifeless. Once you stimulate the flow of blood with a little exercise, however, the opening of vascular channels and nerve pathways will literally charge your muscles with energy.

Don't let your mind talk you into being tired. Ask your

mate or a friend to give you a nudge every time you tell someone how tired you are. Then correct your statement by saying "I feel good and I have plenty of energy." You might be surprised at the results of your optimism.

SUMMARY

1. If you can learn to banish fatigue through healthful living, you'll automatically build youthful health and vigor that will prolong your life.

2. Since fatigue is a symptom that accompanies all types of illness, persons suffering from chronic fatigue should have a medical checkup. About 95 percent of all fatigue complaints, however, stem from bad living habits.

3. Eliminating fatigue will increase your resistance against disease.

4. If your fatigue is unrelieved by sleep and rest, you may have emotional problems that must be dealt with firmly and positively. Don't let fatigue become a mental habit.

5. Take frequent rest breaks during the day so that you can lie down and elevate your legs while you take a couple of deep breaths.

6. If you must sit or stand most of the day, a short walk will stimulate respiration and circulation to aid in preventing fatigue.

7. Nervous fatigue is more serious than physical fatigue, since it can cause all types of illness.

8. Persons who are unhappy with a job that cannot be changed should adopt a hobby or avocation that will satisfy their need to be creative and useful.

9. Lack of exercise, improper diet, inadequate sleep, and other violations of healthful, natural living are common causes of fatigue.

10. Sitting in a rocking chair and rocking at a brisk rate will prevent fatigue by pumping blood through the body.

3

How to Boost Youthfulness by Controlling Your Blood Sugar

If you suffer from fatigue, weakness, headache, irregular heart beat, dizziness, trembling, cold sweats, inability to think, excessive hunger, depression, mental illness, or any of a number of "nervous" ailments for which your doctor can find no cause, you might be suffering from low blood sugar, also called hypoglycemia. This means that your blood does not contain enough glucose to provide fuel for your body. And if it isn't corrected, the wear and tear on your organs and your nervous system is bound to cause premature aging.

Although this condition wasn't demonstrated clinically until 1924, it has been estimated that as many as 30 to 50 million Americans may be suffering from fatigue caused by low blood sugar. Unfortunately, the disorder is rarely recognized or properly treated.

Many persons suffering from hypoglycemia are referred to psychiatrists after undergoing long and fruitless courses of treatment for a variety of vague complaints. Most doctors assume that if they are unable to diagnose a disorder that does not respond to conventional treatment methods, it must be emotional in origin, so they send the patient to a psychiatrist. Many of our complaints *are* emotional in origin; but if you are feeling old, weak, and "run down," it would be a good idea to eliminate low blood sugar as a cause. You can do this by following the instructions in this chapter. Your entire body will benefit, even if your blood sugar is normal. So you have nothing to lose and everything to gain by undergoing the "treatment" as a matter of routine. *Once you have eliminated any chance that you might become a victim of hypoglycemia, you'll be able to get maximum results from your youth-building program.*

WHAT CAUSES HYPOGLYCEMIA?

For the most part, your body gets the sugar it needs from the carbohydrates you eat. When you eat a potato, for example, the starchy portion is converted to a form of sugar that is absorbed through the intestinal wall. Some remains in the blood and some is carried to the liver where it is converted to glycogen and stored for future use as fuel. Your muscles also store glycogen.

The amount of sugar in your blood is controlled by insulin, which is secreted by your pancreas. When there is too much sugar in your blood, your pancreas secretes a little additional insulin. When blood sugar gets too low, your pancreas withholds insulin. A hormone from the adrenal gland then signals the liver to convert enough glycogen to glucose to bring blood sugar back up to normal.

When there is a *deficiency* of insulin, too much sugar may accumulate in the blood and cause diabetes. (Frequent urination and excessive thirst may be early symptoms of diabetes.)

When there is an *excess* of insulin, too much sugar is *removed* from the blood, depriving the body of fuel. In other words, hyperinsulinism causes hypoglycemia, or low blood sugar.

Sudden hunger and weakness accompanied by cold sweat, trembling, and a rapid heart rate are the most outstanding symptoms of low blood sugar. These symptoms can be relieved almost immediately by eating carbohydrates or sweets. Too much sugar in the diet, however, can *cause* low blood sugar! Once you understand how this can happen, you'll be able to prevent the type of fatigue and premature aging caused by a fuel-starved body. This important secret will be revealed to you in this chapter, but first let me tell you about two victims of hypoglycemia.

How One Woman Cured Her Mental Illness

Women between the ages of 30 and 50 seem to be the most common victims of low blood sugar. Improper dieting for figure-control purposes may be the reason. Women who substitute coffee and cigarettes or sweet rolls and coffee for a balanced meal, for example, are likely to suffer from malnutrition as well as hypoglycemia.

A case history in a psychiatrist's notebook tells about Martha B., a 48-year-old woman who suffered from such severe emotional illness that she was repeatedly subjected to electrical shock therapy in an effort to bring her out of a "nervous collapse." The treatment did not help, however, and she was on the verge of committing suicide, when a general practitioner discovered that she had an extremely low blood sugar. A study of her eating habits revealed that she drank huge amounts of coffee and tea each day, both heavily sweetened with sugar. She ate irregularly, and her meals consisted of predominately carbohydrate foods.

When the doctor examined her abdomen, he found that pressure applied to the area just beneath her rib cage on the left side caused pain and spasm of the abdominal muscles.

"All of your trouble may be coming from a bad diet," the doctor told Martha. "Forget about your drugs and pills for a while and let me put you on a special diet."

Martha was placed on a high-protein diet, with several between-meal snacks. She eliminated coffee and tea entirely, and drank fruit juice and skim milk. Even though she ate three meals a day, she lost weight. Best of all, her nerves calmed, her interest in her husband was renewed, and her zest for living returned. In addition to once again being a good wife and a thoughtful mother, she took pride in cooking a good meal and keeping a clean house. For the first time in years, she had energy to spare, even after a long hard day. She looked younger and felt younger—all because of a few simple changes in her diet.

How a Salesman Increased His Energy While Losing Weight

Paul G., a medical equipment salesman, had been complaining of fatigue and weakness for several years. Since he was overweight, his doctors usually recommended a reducing diet after a physical examination failed to reveal any organic disease. Paul found it impossible to stay on the diet while traveling, however, and he was usually so hungry in the middle of the morning and a few hours after dinner that he could not resist between-meal snacks of sandwiches, candy, and soft drinks. If he didn't stop along the road to eat, he would develop a headache that would persist until his next meal.

"I get so hungry," he said, "that I feel as if I'm going to pass out. And I have trouble seeing the road."

Paul was also suffering from attacks of "weak knees," trembling, and cold sweat, which he felt were the result of fear and emotional instability. He had lost confidence in his ability to deal with people. He found it so difficult to concentrate that his business was suffering from inefficient management.

"I guess I had better retire," he said with considerable regret. "At the end of the day, I'm so tired I can hardly make it home. I feel as if I'm going to collapse at any moment. I'm just not well. I must be getting old."

At 50 years of age, Paul looked and felt like an old man.

A series of blood sugar tests revealed that he didn't have enough glucose in his blood to supply the fuel his body needed.

"How can that be?" he asked with astonishment. "I eat plenty of sugar, especially candy."

Like most people, Paul didn't understand the effect that excessive use of sugar can have on the body. By making a simple correction in his eating habits, he experienced a rebirth of strength and energy and, like Martha, *he lost weight.* He returned to his selling job with renewed enthusiasm, and soon found that the day just wasn't long enough to do all the things he wanted to do. The fatigue lines in his face disappeared. He looked ten years younger than he did a year earlier.

THE DIFFERENCE BETWEEN FUNCTIONAL AND ORGANIC HYPOGLYCEMIA

There are several causes of hypoglycemia. All of them can be grouped into two main categories: organic or functional.

Organic hypoglycemia is caused by disease that must be treated by a physician. When the disease is cured, the blood sugar returns to normal and symptoms of hypoglycemia disappear.

Most of the time, however, low blood sugar is *functional* in origin; that is, it's caused by emotional stress, overwork, poor diet, loss of sleep, and other disturbing influences that most of us contend with every day of our life. *Improper diet is the most common cause of hypoglycemia.*

There is a simple way to tell whether your low blood sugar is caused by disease or by a bad diet.

If you can hardly drag yourself out of bed in the morning, and you wake up with headache, fatigue, and other symptoms that are relieved by eating breakfast, you should have a medical checkup. You may be suffering from an organic disease.

If you feel all right in the morning, however, but experience fatigue and other symptoms a few hours *after* eating, you may be suffering from functional hypoglycemia caused by an improper diet. If so, there's a great deal that you can do to help yourself.

HOW IMPROPER DIET LOWERS BLOOD SUGAR

Everyone knows that sugar supplies energy. So what do you do when you feel that you need a little extra energy? Chances are you eat a piece of candy or drink a cup of coffee or a soft drink. This may give you an immediate lift, but if you're a victim of hypoglycemia this may be the worst thing you can do. The concentrated sugar in such products loads the blood with too much glucose. The pancreas is abnormally stimulated, so that too much insulin is released to cope with the excess sugar. As a result, so much sugar is removed from the blood that there is a sudden and drastic *drop* in blood sugar. This causes weakness, hunger, trembling, headache, and other symptoms commonly associated with low blood sugar. Even blackout can occur in severe cases. (Diabetics who take too much insulin experience similar symptoms.)

Each time the blood sugar drops as a result of eating sugar, a recurring hunger or craving for sugar leads the individual back to the candy machine or coffee stand. This keeps building up the blood sugar and then knocking it down, creating a sugar addict with symptoms that defy diagnosis and treatment.

Persons who nibble on sweets all day are usually very fat and always hungry. We've all seen tremendously fat people take time out from work to eat a piece of candy or drink a cola. "I'm just too hungry and too weak to wait until lunch," they say. "I just don't have any energy, and I *crave* sweets."

Many people who voice such complaints literally fan a flame within their bodies when they depend upon sweets for energy. A factory worker who sits on a precarious perch, or an airline pilot who must be alert at all times, cannot afford the risk of developing symptoms of low blood sugar by eating candy between meals.

Not everyone who eats sweets will experience the reaction of low blood sugar. Everyone, however, should avoid excessive use of sugar. Once it becomes established that the individual suffers from functional hypoglycemia, he should eliminate sweets altogether.

According to a survey made by the Department of Agriculture in 1965, consumption of cake, cookies, sweet rolls, and a similar products had increased 65 percent in ten years! This means that a great many people are probably satisfying their appetite with a "quick lunch" of coffee and sweet white-flour products.

Beware of Coffee

Coffee is a favorite rest-break beverage in America. Many people find that a cup of coffee will give them an immediate and stimulating lift. Even tension headache can sometimes be relieved by the caffeine in coffee, which constricts cerebral blood vessels that have been dilated by fatigue and nerve irritation.

Unfortunately, excessive use of coffee, like excessive use of sugar, can lead to low blood sugar in some persons. The caffeine stimulates the adrenal glands, which then release a hormone that causes the liver to release too much sugar into the blood. If the pancreas has been made sensitive by repeated extreme fluctuations in the blood sugar level, it will overreact by releasing too much insulin. This will quickly lower blood sugar to a point far below that needed to supply the body and the brain with adequate oxygen.

Tea and cola drinks also contain caffeine, along with considerable sugar.

HYPOGLYCEMIA AS A CAUSE OF ERRATIC BEHAVIOR

You already know that glucose serves as fuel for the body. But did you know that the brain and the nervous system must have glucose to utilize oxygen? The truth is that the brain runs almost exclusively on sugar.

It shouldn't be hard to imagine what might happen to the brain if there were a sudden and drastic drop in blood sugar. All sorts of erratic behavior might result. The individual may become irritable, angry, moody, depressed, confused, or sleepy. He may even become "mean" enough to commit a crime, even murder. The deficiency of sugar and oxygen in the brain short-circuits nerve centers so that the individual cannot reason clearly or behave rationally. His reaction to his environment cannot be predicted. Some researchers have even tried to link juvenile delinquency with low blood sugar caused by excessive use of sugar and candy.

There's no doubt that too much sugar can contribute to premature aging. Be sure to read Chapter 9 for an explanation of how sugar can deprive the brain and the heart of adequate blood by hardening the arteries.

SUGAR ROBS YOUR BODY OF VITAMIN B

The average American eats more than 100 pounds of white sugar each year. Many eat as much as 300 pounds in one year! So it's safe to say that most of us eat too much sugar. Even the smallest amount of refined sugar in the diet is too much, and it almost always represents extra calories.

It's now well known among nutritionists that thiamine or Vitamin B_1 aids in the assimilation of sugar and starches. When you eat natural carbohydrate, the Vitamin B you need is supplied by the food itself. But when you eat refined sugar or white-flour products, your body must "steal" Vitamin B from your muscles, nerves, and organs. Obviously, if you eat large quantities of refined sugars and starches, you may suffer from a thiamine deficiency that can cause fatigue, nervousness, constipation, and other symptoms.

THE PANCREAS PRESSURE TEST

If you seem to be addicted to sweets and you suffer from any of the symptoms of low blood sugar, try this pancreas pressure test.

Lie on your back so that the muscles of your abdomen will be completely relaxed. Press into the left side of your abdomen, just beneath your ribs, with the fingertips of both hands.

If your pancreas has been overworked by excessive sugar stimulation, it will be tender to light pressure.

Low blood sugar or hypoglycemia can then be confirmed by a series of glucose tolerance tests (supervised by a physician) that will measure the amount of sugar in your blood after drinking glucose solutions.

HOW TO EAT TO CURE AND PREVENT HYPOGLYCEMIA

Whether you suffer from hypoglycemia or not, you should make an effort to eliminate candy, soft drinks, and other sugar-rich foods from your diet. Even if such foods do not trigger an insulin reaction in your body, they may contribute to overweight or to the development of diabetes or atherosclerosis.

A diet that's high in protein and low in carbohydrate is usually prescribed for victims of functional hypoglycemia. Sugar, of course, is a carbohydrate. Refined-flour foods, such as spaghetti, pastries, and white bread, are potent sources of blood sugar.

Everyone can benefit from a diet that's high in protein and low in carbohydrate and fat.

Food Sources of Protein

Each time you eat, you should select predominantly protein foods along with fresh fruits and vegetables. Skim milk, cottage cheese, baked chicken, broiled fish, beans, egg white, nuts, and whole wheat products are rich in protein and low in hard or saturated fat. Fruits and vegetables contain very little protein, but they are rich in vitamins and minerals, and their natural carbohydrate content will supply you with energy without building up your fat stores.

Beef, pork, cheddar cheese, whole milk, and whole milk products are good sources of protein, but, unfortuantely, they are also rich in saturated fat. If you're overweight or over 40, you should cut down on all foods containing animal fat. Chapter 9 will tell you how to do this.

Try to eliminate refined sugar completely. This includes all products made with white sugar. Foods made from white flour should also be eliminated.

You need a small amount of fat in your diet, but it should come from foods that contain unsaturated or soft fat.

Between-Meal Snacks

If you continue to suffer from hunger, weakness, headache, and other symptoms of low blood sugar in spite of high-protein meals, you may need to include between-meal snacks. Fruit, unsweetened orange juice, or cottage cheese and whole wheat wafers are good sources of low-fat energy. Skim milk or peanut butter and crackers will provide long-lasting energy that's slowly absorbed by the intestinal tract. Nuts of all types are also a good source of protein-rich energy, and they're high in unsaturated fat and low in saturated fat.

If you crave sweets, try eating fresh fruits. If this doesn't satisfy your sweet tooth, try dried fruits, such as raisins, dates, apricots, peaches, apple rings, and so on. Get the unsulphured sun-dried type whenever possible. Dried fruits contain proportionately more fructose or fruit sugar than fresh fruits, so they should be eaten in smaller quantities.

Honey is a predigested carbohydrate that's rich in glucose, and it can be absorbed directly into the blood stream for quick energy. Excessive use of honey, however, might trigger an insulin reaction or a fall in blood sugar in some persons.

If you eat properly each day, your liver and your muscles will contain enough stored energy (glycogen) to permit many hours of work or exercise without development of the symptoms of low blood sugar. If you ever do experience weakness and trembling after prolonged exertion, a little honey stirred into a glass of orange juice will quickly replenish your energy stores.

IT COULD BE YOUR NERVES!

Emotional stress can also trigger low blood sugar. Every time you "blow your stack," for example, or when you become emotionally upset, your body secretes adrenalin, which signals the liver to release glucose (from its glycogen stores) in preparing the body for "fight or flight." Since very few of us vent our emotions or anger in actual physical exertion, an accumulation of blood sugar may trigger a massive release of insulin from the pancreas. As a result, so much sugar is removed from the blood that anxiety, trembling, rapid heart rate, and other symptoms of hypoglycemia linger long after an emotional crisis. The blood sugar level can be restored to normal by eating protein foods or natural sweets, but it can be quickly lowered again by another emotional upset.

Try to avoid repeated emotional upsets. When you do face a disturbing situation, try not to "go to pieces" or lose control of your emotions. Remind yourself that you are the master of your nerves, and that you will remain calm no matter what happens. You'll be surprised at how much self-control you have.

There are some sensitive and high-strung persons who are constantly in the throes of emotional stress. The salesman who can't make a sale, the office worker with an unreasonable boss, a struggling young husband with critical inlaws, or a married person with an argumentative or sexually unresponsive mate, for example, may always be "weak and tired." In such cases, fatigue may be largely psychological, but day after day of failure, rejection, or criticism may cause such drastic falls in blood sugar that some actual damage to the nervous system may occur.

I often advise business executives, school teachers, and other persons to work off their anger or frustrations in physical exercise before going home each evening. Punching a bag, jogging around the block, or jumping a rope, for example, will "work off the adrenalin." The exercise will also burn excess blood sugar to prevent overstimulation of the pancreas. Remember, however, that excessive or unaccustomed exertion can burn blood sugar faster than the liver can replace it, especially in untrained persons. So be careful not to overexercise if you want to avoid fatigue caused by depletion of glycogen stores in your muscles.

THE CASE OF THE INSTANT DRUNK

Frank C. was a "social drinker." He didn't keep alcoholic drinks at home, but he would have a few during social or business engagements. One evening during a sales conference, he passed out after having only two drinks.

"Take him home and let him sleep it off," suggested a friend who assumed that Frank was simply intoxicated.

Since Frank was a bachelor, he was transported to his apartment and put to bed. Late the next day, he was still in bed, ill and nearly unconscious. A neighbor finally called a doctor, who reported that Frank was suffering from low blood sugar. He revived him by feeding him glucose through his veins. "Had Frank been left unattended much longer," the doctor said, "he might have died."

Frank's trouble was not drunkenness, but hypoglycemia. It seems that he had been too busy to take time out to eat on that particular day, and when he filled his stomach with cocktails, the reaction of the alcohol on his body caused a drastic drop in an already low blood sugar. He lost consciousness because his brain was being deprived of adequate glucose and oxygen.

Always eat before drinking alcohol—if you drink at all. When you have guests "in for a drink," serve cheese and crackers along with the drinks.

If someone in your group becomes "clobbered" by alcohol, feed him a glass of orange juice mixed with a tablespoonful of honey. This will restore his blood sugar and help to sober him up. Forget about black coffee. The caffeine in the coffee might cause a further drop in blood sugar by stimulating the adrenal glands.

Chronic alcoholics must often have medical help in restoring their blood sugar. The liver of an alcoholic may be so infiltrated with fat that it cannot store adequate glycogen. As a result, a deficiency of glucose in the blood creates a craving for sugar that is satisfied by drinking.

SUMMARY

1. Excessive use of refined sugar can *lower* blood sugar by overstimulating your pancreas.

2. A deficiency of glucose in the blood deprives the body of adequate fuel. It also deprives the brain and the nervous system of adequate oxygen.

3. Low blood sugar, also called hypoglycemia, can cause a great variety of symptoms along with fatigue and hunger.

4. Persons who suffer from hypoglycemia should cut down on carbohydrates and eat predominately protein foods. Refined sugar and white-flour products should be eliminated altogether.

5. Between-meal snacks of skim milk, fresh fruit, fruit juice, cheese, or nuts will relieve symptoms of low blood sugar. Do not eat candy or drink coffee or soda pop between meals.

6. The caffeine in coffee, tea, and cola drinks stimulates the adrenal glands, which trigger hypoglycemia.

7. Never drink alcohol on an empty stomach. Sober up or combat hangovers with orange juice and honey rather than black coffee.

8. Try to maintain a tranquil mind. Emotional stress and strain is a common cause of nervous fatigue, and it can trigger low blood sugar through the adrenal glands.

9. Hypoglycemia caused by improper diet usually develops a couple of hours after eating starches or sweets.

10. If symptoms of low blood sugar persist after observing the dietary recommendations outlined in this chapter, your trouble may be organic rather than dietary or functional.

4

How to Eat Natural Foods for a Long, Youthful Life

Back in the early 1900's, Dr. Alexis Carrel withdrew the blood of an invalid 18-year-old dog and replaced the serum portion with an artificial solution of the same composition. The results were miraculous. The dog began running and barking like a young pup, and he grew new hair. Even his interest in sex was revived.

Dr. Carrel also kept cell fragments from the heart of a chicken embryo alive for 34 years in a special nutritive solution. He terminated the experiment with the opinion that the tissue could be kept alive indefinitely if someone bothered to maintain the solution.

"Tissue cells are essentially immortal," wrote Dr. Carrel. "Give cells all the essential nutrition they need, remove all wastes and poisons, and they can be kept alive indefinitely."

In another interesting experiment designed to prove that the chemical composition of the blood had something to do with aging, Dr. Carrel withdrew blood serum from an "old" chicken and put it in a solution that contained live tissue. As he expected, the growth of the tissue was retarded and the aging process was accelerated.

Science has not yet found out how to completely eliminate the toxins generated by living tissue in a living body. It is possible, however, to postpone the aging process by enriching the blood with the nutrients of carefully chosen foods and then taking steps to stimulate the circulation of blood.

You'll learn in Chapter 6 how to improve your circulation so that you can help your system neutralize the toxins released by the tissue cells. And you'll learn in Chapters 5 and 7 how to speed elimination of waste products with improved bowel and breathing habits. But you must first learn how to supply your body with the nutrients it needs to build healthy tissue.

DON'T WAIT FOR A YOUTH PILL

Your corner drug store does not yet sell a "youth pill" that will grow hair on a bald head or send an octogenarian on a honeymoon, but at least one medical researcher has developed a "youth drug" that he claims will extend the life span indefinitely—and a major drug company has invested in his theory.

Once the chemical process of aging has been completely analyzed, it's not too farfetched to predict the development of a youth serum that will prolong life. But chances are the instructions on the bottle will read: "Effective only if you observe the basic laws of healthy living." So don't just do nothing and wait around for a pill that will give you a few extra years of life. Your health depends upon how well you take care of your body *now.*

There will never be a youth serum that will prevent disease caused by bad living habits. People today are dying of *disease* rather than old age. So even if there were a serum or a pill that would prolong life, you'd have to have a healthy body to take advantage of it.

NUTRITION MOST IMPORTANT

Lord Bacon once wrote that "Diet well ordered bears the greatest part in the prolongation of life." He was right—then as now.

Rest, sleep, exercise, recreation, emotional tranquility, and other factors are all important in building youthful health, but the average person probably damages his health most with bad eating habits. Heart disease, the nation's No. 1 killer, for example, is now believed to stem primarily from too much sugar and fat in the diet.

Refined and artificial foods are robbing our bodies of important vitamins and minerals and poisoning our tissues with chemical additives. The result is that resistance to infection is lowered, and a breakdown of tissue causes disease and premature aging.

It's never too late to correct a bad diet. But the younger you are when you begin to pay attention to your eating habits the better the results in building a body that will last 100 years or longer.

"Good eating habits in early life will bring us vigorous maturity," says the Department of Agriculture in its year-book *Food*. "A continuance of them will extend our years of usefulness and delay—and, in some instances, even prevent—the appearance of many of the so-called characteristics of old age."

Begin with a Balanced Diet

Although certain vitamins and minerals may be singled out as having some special effect in postponing the aging process, it's important to remember that your body needs *all* of the various food elements in order to be healthy. Some vitamins and minerals cannot even be absorbed without the presence of other important elements or enzymes. Calcium is essential in building bones, for example, but it does so with the assistance of phosphorus, protein, and Vitamins A, C, and D.

A deficiency in any vitamin or mineral, or inadequate protein, carbohydrate, or fat, can cause premature aging and fatigue. For this reason, it's important to *make sure that you eat a variety of natural, wholesome foods in a balanced diet each day.*

Always try to select one or more foods from these four groups every time you eat: (1) milk and milk products; (2) meat, poultry, fish, or eggs; (3) whole grain bread or cereal; (4) fruits and vegetables.

Natural Foods Best

There is no longer any doubt among nutrition experts that natural, unrefined foods are best for good health. Observation of the eating habits of both animals and humans has shown conclusively that health and longevity are related to food. The normal life span of rats, for example, has been *doubled* by keeping them on wholesome vitamin-rich foods. And it has been *shortened* by placing them on a diet of white bread, margarine, sweet tea, white sugar, jam, preserved meat, and overcooked vegetables. In fact, rats on such a diet have developed many of the diseases that now shorten the life of the average American.

A study of the Hunza tribe in India by Dr. Robert McCarrison back in 1918 has provided us with an example of the kind of diet that builds youthful health and vigor. These people, untouched by civilization, were long-lived, vigorous in youth and in old age, and remarkably free of disease.

"During my period of association with these people," said Dr. McCarrison, "I never saw a case of asthenic dyspepsia, or gastric or duodenal ulcer, appendicitis, mucous colitis, or of cancer."

The diet of the Hunzas consisted of flat bread made of whole wheat flour lightly smeared with butter, sprouted legumes, fresh raw carrots, raw cabbage, unpasteurized whole milk and soured milk, a small ration of meat with bones once a week, and an abundance of water.

YOU CAN EAT TO PREVENT PREMATURE AGING

There is considerable evidence that the normal life span can be lengthened by altering the diet. The primary object of the material in this chapter, however, is to help you prevent premature aging and disease caused by a deficiency in certain important food elements. You can eat for pleasure as well as for health, and live longer as a result, by eating the foods supplied by nature.

HOW TO GET ALL THE CALCIUM YOU NEED TO STAY YOUNG

When Dr. C. Ward Crampton presented his report to the New York State Joint Legislative Committee on Nutrition in 1947, he informed the group that the American diet was deficient in calcium. He also said that *calcium poverty is one common cause of aging that can be corrected!*

In Chapter 2, I quoted a Department of Agriculture survey that revealed that Americans are now more deficient in calcium than ever before.

The Many Roles of Calcium

About 99 percent of the total amount of calcium in your body is in your bones and teeth. The remaining one percent is essential to the functioning of every cell in your body. It's necessary for the normal clotting of blood, for the functioning of important enzymes, and *for controlling the passage of fluids through the walls of tissue cells.* Your muscles, nerves, and heart cannot function normally when blood calcium is low.

When there is a deficiency of calcium in the diet, the body draws enough from the bones of the spine and pelvis to sustain life. But if this goes on for very long, the vertebrae become porous and brittle, and impaired function of the tissue cells permits the accumulation of toxins that hasten the aging process.

In your effort to build youthful health and vigor, you should try to get *more* than enough calcium to maintain the strength of your bones and the health of your tissue cells.

What About Milk?

Everyone knows that milk contains a great deal of calcium. There is some difference in opinion, however, about the nutritional value of milk. Some people believe that destruction of the enzyme phosphatase in pasteurized milk makes it impossible for the body to absorb the calcium. Others believe that an excessive amount of calcium from milk can result in calcium deposits in arthritic joints. Neither of these beliefs is entirely true.

It's true that pasteurization destroys the enzymes in milk, along with ten percent of its Vitamin B_1 and 30 percent of its Vitamin C. But according to the Department of Agriculture, one quart of whole milk supplies more than the usual calcium requirement, as well as two-thirds of the daily phosphorus requirement, one-third of the Vitamin A requirement, and a full quota of riboflavin. In fact, most nutritionists maintain that *it is difficult to get the amount of calcium you need without using milk in some form each day.*

Whatever nutrients may be lacking in pasteurized milk can be supplied in other foods in the diet.

If you don't want to drink pasteurized milk, drink *certified* raw milk or none at all. There are many dangerous bacteria that thrive in improperly prepared milk.

You don't have to worry about getting too much calcium from milk. The amount of calcium your body absorbs will be governed largely by its needs. Your kidneys will excrete the calcium your body doesn't use.

Warning for Ulcer Patients

If you have an ulcer or "acid indigestion" and you drink a great deal of milk, you should be cautious about taking antacids or baking soda. Use of alkalies with milk will permit the absorption of a form of calcium that your body cannot use or eliminate. The blood stream will then be forced to dump the "dead" calcium into joints and tissues where it forms irritating deposits.

Other Sources of Calcium

If you don't drink milk, try to include some milk products in your diet each day. *Unprocessed cheeses* of all kinds are rich in calcium. If you're on a low-fat diet, you can eat *cottage cheese* or *yogurt.* In addition to being rich in calcium, cultured yogurt contains a type of bacteria that will aid digestion and elimination (see Chapter 5). *Buttermilk* is also low in fat, and it's just as rich in calcium as sweet milk.

Don't make the mistake of flavoring your milk with cocoa. This would combine oxalic acid with calcium to prevent the calcium from being fully absorbed and utilized. If you must drink flavored milk, try using *carob powder.* This delicious, naturally sweet powder tastes very much like chocolate, and it's rich in vitamins and minerals.

Powdered skim milk can be added to puddings, bread, ice cream, and other home-prepared foods to increase their calcium content.

Vegetables Also Contain Calcium

Many foods outside the milk group contain a small amount of calcium. *Green leafy vegetables,* for example, contribute a fair amount of calcium in a balanced diet. Spinach, beet greens, chard, and rhubarb, however, contain oxalic acid, which prevents absorption of the calcium. The calcium in spinach is excreted by the bowels. So don't follow "Popeye's" example in the newspaper comic strip and eat only spinach.

Almonds, oysters, dried beans, and dark molasses contain relatively large amounts of calcium.

Special Calcium Supplements

Persons who use little or no milk products should probably add *bone meal* to their diet. In powder or tablet form, this natural supplement supplies calcium along with plenty of phosphorus and Vitamin D to facilitate its absorption and use.

Egg shell powder is also a good source of calcium. You can extract the calcium from a whole egg shell by soaking it overnight in a little lemon juice. The acid will dissolve the calcium so that you may add the solution to your favorite fruit or vegetable juice for a calcium-rich drink. (It might be a good idea to boil the egg shell before soaking it, just to make sure that it's free of germs.)

The Special Needs of the Elderly

The older a person becomes, the more likely he is to be deficient in calcium. The reason, of course, is that *old people tend to have less hydrochloric acid in their stomach, and acid is necessary for the absorption of calcium.* This may be one reason why so many elderly persons suffer from osteoporosis of the spine, a condition in which the vertebrae become thin and brittle from lack of adequate calcium. The tissue cells, also starved for calcium, age prematurely because of their inability to exchange wastes for nutrients. (Remember that calcium is necessary for the ionic balance that permits the passage of elements *through* the walls of tissue cells.)

Many doctors recommend additional calcium for all their elderly patients, along with phosphorus and Vitamin D. Highly concentrated calcium supplements should probably also include magnesium, since excess calcium can result in urinary loss of magnesium. Try to get the calcium you need from natural foods, so that you'll get all the other food elements you need in proper combinations. Your bones will store the calcium you need for use in emergencies.

Protein is also needed in building the framework of bones. Milk is a good source of protein, but you'll need to include meat or eggs. Most protein foods also contain phosphorus, which will help you absorb calcium. Always include some vegetables or milk with your meat so that there'll be a balance between calcium and phosphorus.

Exercise Strengthens Bones

When no stress is placed on bones, they lose calcium, no matter how much milk you drink. The more exercise you take, the more calcium your bones will store and the stronger they'll be.

VITAMIN C–THE BEAUTY AND YOUTH VITAMIN

Vitamin C is so important in building youthful health that it is sometimes called "the beauty and youth vitamin." It is unfortunate that it is so commonly deficient in the average American diet.

"Cement" for Tissue Cells

Vitamin C or ascorbic acid supplies a "cement" that holds the tissue cells together, and it strengthens blood vessels and capillaries. When there is a deficiency of Vitamin C, tissue sags and loses its firmness, resistance to infection is greatly reduced, and wounds heal slowly. In pronounced deficiencies, the gums will be sore, and the body bruises and bleeds easily. Bleeding from the wall of a small blood vessel may even originate a clot that could cause a fatal heart attack.

Since the aging process seems to begin with a breakdown of connective tissue and collagen and a deterioration of the walls of tissue cells, it seems likely that an increased amount of Vitamin C in the diet would greatly aid in building firm and youthful tissue. There's one thing for sure: A *deficiency* in Vitamin C is bound to contribute to premature aging. And we know that Vitamin C must be available for the regeneration of collagen.

A deficiency severe enough to cause scurvy is rare, since just about everyone eats Irish potatoes and a few popular vegetables that contain small amounts of Vitamin C. No one knows exactly how much of this vitamin the average person needs to maintain the best health possible. But studies of blood plasma indicate that many people have *less* than the amount of Vitamin C known to be essential in maintaining what has been called "good health."

You Need Vitamin C Every Day for Youthfulness

The body does not store Vitamin C for future use. If you should absorb more of this vitamin than your tissues can use on any given day, the excess will be eliminated through your kidneys. This means that you should eat something containing Vitamin C at each meal. It might be a good idea to eat something rich in Vitamin C between meals.

Keeping your tissues *saturated* with Vitamin C may be very important in keeping your flesh youthful. *Lab experiments with animals have revealed that the younger the animal the greater the concentration of Vitamin C in its tissues.* And according to the U.S. Department of Agriculture, "The higher concentration of Vitamin C in young tissue than in old and the high concentration in actively multiplying cells and tissue indicate that Vitamin C must be present where tissue is formed or regenerated."

The body is constantly breaking down old tissue and replacing it with new. In order to make sure that degeneration does not exceed regeneration, try to get all the Vitamin C you can from fresh, natural foods—the more the better.

Natural Food Sources of Vitamin C

Citrus fruits, tomatoes, and cabbage are among the best and most common sources of Vitamin C. Many fruits and vegetables contain generous amounts of this vitamin. A handful of fresh strawberries will supply enough Vitamin C to meet the basic needs of the body for one day. Green peppers and parsley contain *more* Vitamin C than is normally found in citrus fruits. Sweet and Irish potatoes are fairly good sources.

With a great variety of fruits, vegetables, melons, and berries in a balanced diet, the average person can get all the Vitamin C he needs to stay youthful and healthy. *Be sure to eat some fresh fruit every day.*

How You Lose Vitamin C

Vitamin C is more easily destroyed than most vitamins. Since it is water soluble, much of it is lost when vegetables are soaked in water. Exposure to heat during cooking also accounts for much loss. Even light and oxygen can destroy Vitamin C when fruits and vegetables are harvested and stored. Stress and nervous tension seem to destroy Vitamin C in the tissues.

How to Get More Vitamin C

The best way to get the Vitamin C you need is to eat fruits and vegetables *raw* whenever possible—and the fresher they are the better.

Fruits, of course, should always be eaten raw. If the skin is edible, wash the fruit with mild soap and water (to remove oily pesticides) and eat the skin along with the fruit. If the fruit has been dyed or waxed, the skin should be discarded.

It's much better to eat the meat of a fruit than to squeeze it for juice. In addition to providing roughage for your intestinal tract, fruit pulp contains Vitamin P, which aids Vitamin C in strengthening blood vessels and capillaries.

Cooking Hints

In order to reduce the exposure of vegetables to heat and

water, they should be cooked in as short a time as possible. If you have any "waterless" cookware, you can cook your vegetables in steam. Otherwise, put just enough water in the bottom of the pot to prevent scorching the vegetables, cover the pot with a heavy lid, and then cook them until they're just tender enough to eat. If there is any water left in the pot, don't throw it away. You can boil it down and use it as a sauce.

Remember that the more of the vegetable that's exposed to air, the greater the loss of Vitamin C to oxygen. So don't cut your vegetables into small pieces. Cut them just large enough to permit cooking and then try to avoid breaking them into small pieces. When vegetables are boiled to a mush, the small amount of Vitamin C that survives the heat is in the cooking water, which is usually poured down the drain.

Always serve vegetables just as soon after cooking as possible. Keep them covered until they are placed on the table, ready to eat.

There are many vegetables that are very tasty when eaten raw. Whenever you cook such vegetables, always put a little aside to serve raw in salads.

A Warning for Smokers

The nicotine from one cigarette destroys the amount of Vitamin C you get from one orange. If you smoke several cigarettes each day, you need a great deal more Vitamin C than a nonsmoker would need.

The best thing to do is to quit smoking—and for many reasons other than loss of Vitamin C. If you just cannot break the habit, you may have to seek concentrated sources of Vitamin C in order to saturate your tissues without eating a crate of oranges every day.

Beware of Alkalizers

Vitamin C is also destroyed by alkaline solutions. Persons

who get into the habit of taking baking soda or antacids may not be able to absorb enough Vitamin C to keep their tissues youthful and healthy.

Special Vitamin C Supplements You Can Make at Home

If you eat fresh fruits and vegetables each day, you won't have to take vitamin pills. But if you feel that you need additional Vitamin C, you can get more than enough from a few home-prepared natural supplements, namely rose hip extract and bean sprouts.

How to Prepare Rose Hip Extract

Rose hips, the seed pods that remain after the rose sheds its petals, are extremely rich in Vitamin C. They are richest during the month of October, when they are bright red in color. Extract from rose hips is 10 to 100 times as rich in Vitamin C as fresh orange juice!

Place the gathered rose hips in a refrigerator and leave them there until they are chilled. This will destroy the enzymes that might react with the Vitamin C during preparation of the extract.

Remove all stems and blossom ends and wash the rose hips very briefly by running faucet water over them for a second or two.

Boil 1½ cups of water for each cup of rose hips. Then add chopped or mashed rose hips (preferably liquified in a blender) and let the mixture simmer for 15 minutes in a sealed pot.

Keep the mixture covered and let it stand for 24 hours in a refrigerator.

The next day, strain the extract and bring it to a boil. After it cools, add two tablespoons of lemon juice for each pint of extract, seal in glass jars, and store in a refrigerator.

Be sure to use glass or stainless steel containers when

preparing the extract. Contact with iron or copper utensils will destroy the Vitamin C.

Add one tablespoonful of rose hip extract to each glass of fruit or vegetable juice you drink, each day.

If you don't want to bother with preparing your own extract, or if rose hips aren't available to you, you can buy rose hips in powder or tablet form in any health food store.

How to Grow Your Own Bean Sprouts

Most peas, beans, seeds, peanuts, and grains contain some Vitamin C, but when they begin to sprout their Vitamin C content increases tremendously. They are also rich in the "living" elements you need to build a youthful body.

Sprouts are delicious, and may be eaten alone or in salads. It's best to eat them raw whenever possible, especially in salads, but they may be cooked in the same way you cook any other vegetable. Chinese cooks have been using bean sprouts for centuries. So have the healthy Hunza tribes in India.

Growing sprouts can be fun. It's fascinating to watch a plant spring from a seed or bean. When you first begin growing sprouts, use only a few beans to begin with. Until you have experimented enough to learn how to get the best results, some of your beans may spoil or turn sour before they've sprouted adequately.

Towel technique of growing sprouts: Warmth and moisture with adequate drainage and ventilation are essential in sprouting any seed or legume. You can get fairly good results by placing beans between two Turkish towels that have been laid over a screen or a broiling tray that has drainage slots. Place the tray on a sink apron and then pour warm water over the towels several times a day to moisten and wash the sprouts. After two or three days at room temperature, the beans should be well sprouted.

Always soak dried peas, beans, or seeds overnight in warm

water before attempting to sprout them. This will soften the kernal and speed sprouting. Be sure to use enough water to allow for swelling of large beans. Your local seed store can supply you with fertile dried beans that will be sure to sprout.

Soybeans: Probably the most nutritious beans you can eat are soybeans, and the dried variety sprout very quickly. The Vitamin C content of soybean sprouts can be increased even more by covering them with a moist cloth and storing them in a refrigerator for a few days.

If you plan to store or freeze the sprouts for lcnger than one week, you can preserve their Vitamin C content by first blanching or boiling them for two minutes to destroy the bean's enzymes.

The flower pot method: After you've soaked the beans overnight, put them in a two-quart flower pot that has been lined with cheese cloth. Sprinkle them with warm water and then cover the pot with a moist wash cloth. Pour water over the beans several times a day. The hole in the bottom of the pot will provide adequate drainage and ventilation.

VITAMIN B COMPLEX IS ALSO IMPORTANT

There are several vitamins in the B complex group, and you need all of them. One does not work without the other.

Thiamine, or Vitamin B_1, is the B vitamin that's most likely to be deficient in the American diet. Like Vitamin C, it is easily destroyed by heat and water during cooking.

Whole wheat is a good source of thiamine; but when wheat is processed, most of the thiamine is milled out. And since this vitamin plays an important role in the metabolism of carbohydrate, excessive use of sugar, pastries, and unenriched white-flour products robs the body of the Vitamin B it needs for a healthy nervous system.

A deficiency of thiamine also allows pyruvic acid to accumulate in the tissues. This by-product of incomplete carbohydrate metabolism can cause fatigue and nervousness that will make you feel twice as old as you really are. You may also suffer from constipation, depression, apathy, numbness, and all sorts of nervous and emotional symptoms.

Milk, eggs, meat, fruit, and vegetables contribute fair amounts of thiamine in a balanced diet. Lean pork, dried beans and peas, and wheat germ are good sources. *Brewer's yeast contains all the B vitamins,* as well as many other important vitamins and minerals.

Riboflavin, or Vitamin B_2, is another water-soluble vitamin that is deficient in many diets. It is not destroyed by heat as Vitamins C and B_1 are, but it is destroyed by sunlight. Pasteurizing milk, for example, does not reduce its riboflavin content very much, but if a bottle of milk is left sitting on a sunny porch there is a rapid loss of the vitamin. This is one reason why milk should be stored in dark bottles in a dark refrigerator.

Milk, meat, cheese, eggs, green leafy vegetables, and whole wheat products are good sources of riboflavin. Just be careful not to "wash out" your meat and vegetables by boiling them in water.

Riboflavin will help your body use all the other B vitamins. The first symptom of a deficiency may be a chronically sore tongue.

The Other B Vitamins

If you eat foods containing the first two B vitamins, chances are you'll get all the other vitamins in the group. Strict vegetarians are sometimes deficient in the important blood-building Vitamin B_{12}, since vegetables do not contain significant amounts of this vitamin. You'll learn more about this in Chapter 8.

Some members of the B complex group, especially those from vegetable sources (cholin and inositol), help to prevent the accumulation of hard fat inside your arteries. *Wheat germ, brewer's yeast, and dark molasses* are good sources of vegetable-type B vitamins.

A Warning for Drinkers

Alcohol destroys Vitamin B, especially thiamine. It is well known that many alcoholics suffer from a Vitamin B deficiency that must be corrected by injections.

If you eat properly, and drink alcohol only occasionally, you probably won't suffer a deficiency. But if you have more than two or three drinks a week, you'd better include a few brewer's yeast tablets in your diet.

VITAMIN A CAN PROLONG YOUR LIFE

Like all vitamins, Vitamin A plays an important role in keeping your body youthful and vigorous. In fact, Dr. Henry C. Sherman, professor emeritus of Columbia University, has said that man could add ten years to his prime of life by eating four times the amount of Vitamin A recommended for the average person.

Since Vitamin A can be stored in the body, an excessive amount of this vitamin from pills or artificially prepared sources can have toxic effects. For this reason, you should try to get your Vitamin A from such natural foods as liver, butter, egg yolk, cheese, and whole milk. If you're on a low-cholesterol diet and you cannot eat these foods, it might be a good idea to add a little fish liver oil to your diet. But don't take more than recommended on the label of the bottle.

Vitamin A is normally found only in foods of animal origin. The carotene in yellow and green vegetables, however, can be converted into Vitamin A in the liver. So be sure to eat plenty of vegetables. And don't throw away the outer dark green leaves of cabbage and other vegetables; they're rich in both carotene and Vitamin C.

Lack of adequate Vitamin A in your diet will lower your

resistance against infection. Much of the protection offered by the skin and the mucous membranes lining the cavities of the body depends upon getting adequate amounts of this vitamin from both animal and vegetable sources. Night blindness can also result from a pronounced deficiency.

DON'T FORGET VITAMIN D

Vitamin D is a fat-soluble vitamin that's frequently deficient in persons who use mineral oil laxatives. This vitamin is not widely distributed in the foods we eat, so you may have to make a special effort to get all you need to maintain a youthful body.

Salt-water fish, liver, and egg yolk contain Vitamin D. So does most commercially bottled milk. But fish liver oil and bone meal are the only rich food sources. You can enrich vegetable oil with Vitamin D by exposing it to the sun's rays in a flat, open pan. You may then add the oil—preferably corn oil or wheat germ oil—to your salads.

The ultraviolet rays of the sun convert an oil in the skin to Vitamin D. Try to expose some portion of your body to unfiltered sunlight each day. Window glass, smog, and dust filter out and absorb the important ultraviolet rays.

Why You Shouldn't Take Vitamin D Pills

Don't take Vitamin D pills unless your doctor prescribes them. If you do take a commercial vitamin, don't take any more than recommended on the bottle's label. Too much artificial Vitamin D can result in absorption of too much calcium, which can cause gastrointestinal trouble, hardened arteries, and even death.

If you get plenty of exposure to sunlight, you probably do not need any extra Vitamin D. But if you're the indoor type, or if you work at night and sleep during the day, you should probably add a little bone meal or fish liver oil to your diet.

A deficiency in Vitamin D results in a deficiency in

calcium and phosphorus, which can weaken nerves, muscles, and tissue cells as well as bones and teeth. The bones, however, show the most obvious results of a Vitamin D deficiency. Children develop rickets, and adults develop osteomalacia. In both cases, the bones become soft and deformed. Many "old" people suffer from soft bones that could be corrected with a little sunlight, bone meal, and exercise.

VITAMIN E—THE NEW YOUTH VITAMIN

Doctors have known about Vitamin E for a long time. But only in recent years have they become fully aware of its importance in building superior health.

Here are some of the functions of this valuable vitamin: (1) improves glandular health and increases production of hormones to prolong youth and increase the life span, (2) improves heart action, (3) increases efficiency of muscles, (4) reduces body's need for oxygen, (5) prevents oxidation of Vitamin A and essential fatty acids, (6) protects blood cells, (7) prevents abnormal clotting of blood to cut down on heart attacks, and (8) slows the aging process by preventing oxidation of tissues.

Obviously, you cannot afford to have even the slightest deficiency in Vitamin E. Fortunately, this fat-soluble vitamin is widely distributed in foods of both plant and animal origin, and there is no loss in cooking. If your diet includes fresh fruits, vegetables, milk, whole-grain cereals, meat, and eggs, you'll probably get adequate amounts of Vitamin E.

One leading physician, however, maintains that milling of grains has deprived Americans of so much Vitamin E that the diet should be supplemented with at least one tablespoonful of wheat germ oil—or some other vegetable oil, such as corn oil—each day for superior nutrition. Vitamin E from natural food sources is nontoxic, so you don't have to worry about getting too much.

Lettuce is a good source of Vitamin E, as well as seeds and nuts. Men who want to increase their intake of Vitamin E for reproductive purposes should try eating pumpkin seeds, which contain a hormone-like substance which protects the prostate gland.

VITAMIN F—THE HEART AND ARTERY VITAMIN

The essential unsaturated fatty acids are "soft fats" that prevent hard fat from accumulating in the arteries. As a group, they are called Vitamin F. Chapter 9, "How to Make Your Heart Last 100 Youthful Years or Longer," will tell you everything you need to know about this new vitamin group.

VITAMIN K CAN BE DESTROYED BY DRUGS

Vitamin K is essential for the clotting of blood and for normal liver function. Your intestinal tract can manufacture this vitamin, and it is so widely distributed in a variety of foods that you are not likely to suffer a deficiency.

Green leafy vegetables, tomatoes, egg yolk, and liver are good sources of Vitamin K. Fortunately, this vitamin is not affected by ordinary cooking procedures.

Since Vitamin K must be absorbed in the intestinal tract in the presence of bile, you might not absorb enough of this vitamin if you have a gall bladder or intestinal disorder. Prolonged treatment with sulfa drugs or antibiotics can also result in a deficiency.

Excessive use of aspirin interferes with the clotting of blood and probably destroys Vitamin K—or at least interferes with its absorption. Surgeons have discovered that some patients who suffer from hemorrhage following surgery have been overdosed with aspirin.

Drugs can save lives and relieve pain when they are properly used. But when used unnecessarily, they can do a great deal of harm. So don't take drugs unless you have to, and only then if they are prescribed by a physician.

Like all the other fat-soluble vitamins, Vitamin K can be washed out of the intestinal tract with mineral oil or undigested cooking grease. Try to avoid excessive use of fried foods.

YOUR BODY FRAMEWORK IS MADE OF PROTEIN

Protein forms the framework for construction of every cell in your body. Your muscles are made almost entirely of protein. So are your fingernails and your hair.

Since old and worn-out cells in your body are constantly being replaced by new cells, you must have protein every day of your life to be in the best of health.

All protein is made up of amino acids. About 22 of them are known to be essential in human nutrition. Your body can manufacture all but eight of them; these you must get by eating certain types of foods.

How to Get the Essential Amino Acids

Foods containing all eight of the essential amino acids are known as first class or complete protein foods. Vegetables contain varying amounts of the different amino acids, but their protein is usually incomplete. This means that you cannot depend upon vegetables alone for an adequate supply of protein. If all eight of the essential amino acids are not present when your body absorbs them, they cannot be used to build tissue.

Meat, fish, and poultry are the best sources of protein, since they supply amino acids in the same combinations found in our tissues. Many "vegetarians" who do not eat meat get most of their amino acids from milk, eggs, and cheese, which are very rich in complete protein.

If you want to get a larger part of your protein from vegetable sources, you can increase your intake of brewer's yeast, soybean products, wheat germ and whole wheat products, peas and beans, peanuts, and sunflower seeds. These foods contain complete protein, but they may be weak in one or more of the essential amino acids. Combined with some other food of animal origin, however, they can form adequate first class protein. *Soybeans* are rich in complete protein, and they compare favorably with meat.

It takes a great deal of food knowledge to select foods from plant sources alone in combining the essential amino acids to form a complete protein. I wouldn't recommend that you try it without help from someone trained in nutrition.

The older you become, the more protein you'll need to repair your aging bones and tissues. But if your doctor tells you to cut down on saturated fat, you'll have to select your foods carefully. Chapter 9 will tell you how to get your protein from foods containing little or no hard fat.

YOU NEED CARBOHYDRATE FOR ENERGY

Carbohydrates supply most of the fuel your body uses for energy. When there is too much carbohydrate in the diet, it is stored in the tissues as fat. Just about everyone who is overweight eats too much carbohydrate, especially the refined variety. Sugar and white-flour products, for example, are highly concentrated carbohydrates, and they are far too plentiful on the American dinner table.

If you have a little flab around the middle, you could probably get rid of it simply by eliminating refined foods. (See Chapter 11 for an effective, effortless reducing program.) Most natural foods contain some carbohydrate, but they are not as concentrated as processed foods. One chocolate bar, for example, contains as much sugar as a dozen apples. Yet, one apple will satisfy the appetite more readily than a dozen chocolate bars. This is one reason why very few people build up excessive fat stores by eating natural foods.

Don't ever attempt to reduce by going on a pure protein

diet. Your body can burn protein and fat for energy, but if there is not enough carbohydrate in the diet there may be some harmful effects. Protein should be used to repair and rebuild tissue cells and to form important enzymes. When some of your daily protein intake must be burned for energy, your muscles and organs may be deprived of the amino acids they need to be strong and healthy. Furthermore, when the body is forced to burn fat in the absence of carbohydrate, there may be an accumulation of harmful acids in the blood. Any diabetic can tell you what happens when the body is unable to burn carbohydrate for energy.

So while most of us should reduce our carbohydrate intake, it should not be cut off entirely. If you eat a balanced diet including the use of fresh fruits and vegetables, you'll get all the carbohydrate you need.

BALANCING FAT FOR GOOD BODY CHEMISTRY

Fat can also supply energy, but not as readily as carbohydrate. Although fat must be reduced to a minimum in the diet of the average person, a certain amount of fat is necessary for good health. The essential fatty acids, which cannot be manufactured by the body, must be supplied by vegetable oils.

When there is no fat of any type in your intestinal tract, the fat soluble vitamins (A, D, E, & K) cannot be absorbed and used by the body. Fortunately, these vitamins are usually found in foods that contain fat or oil.

Your body can manufacture fat from carbohydrate, but this does not supply the essential fatty acids you need to keep hard fat from clogging your arteries.

WHAT ABOUT MINERALS?

Minerals are also important in building youthful health and vigor. If you eat a balanced diet containing all the essential vitamins and amino acids, you'll automatically get the minerals you need. You should, however, make a special effort to make sure that your diet contains foods rich in *calcium, phosphorus, iron, and iodine.* This will leave no doubt that your mineral supply is more than adequate.

You have already learned how to increase your calcium and phosphorus intake. Chapter 8, "How to Build Rich, Red Blood for Youthful Health," will tell you how to increase your intake of iron.

Special Sources of Iodine

Iodine is normally found in small amounts in vegetables. But in some sections of the country, around the Great Lakes and the Rocky Mountains, for example, where soil and water are deficient in iodine, the diet must be supplemented with iodized salt or seafood. All seafoods, both plant and animal, are rich in iodine.

A deficiency in iodine results in enlargement of the thyroid gland. Since this gland plays an important role in regulating body metabolism, a disturbance in its function can speed up the life processes and "burn out" the body prematurely. Or a slow-down might occur, which could shorten your life by making your body fat and·sluggish.

If you use *iodized salt* in a balanced diet, you are probably getting adequate iodine. But you should try to eat sea food at least once a week. It might be a good idea to occasionally eat a little *dried kelp* (seaweed) for iodine insurance. *Sea salt* is also rich in iodine.

You can't get too much iodine from natural foods. Try to eat a variety of foods taken from the sea—for superior nutrition as well as for good eating.

SUMMARY

1. To stay young and healthy, tissue cells must have a free-flowing exchange of toxins for nutrients.

2. Calcium and Vitamin C are the most common deficiencies in the diet of the aging American.

3. In addition to eating a balanced diet to assure an adequate intake of all the food elements that are known to be essential to health, you should make a special effort to eat milk products and fresh raw fruits each day.

4. Cook your vegetables just enough to make them tender. Try to avoid boiling your meats and vegetables in water. Eat some of your vegetables raw whenever possible.

5. Remember that smoking reduces the amount of Vitamin C in your blood. Alcohol destroys Vitamin B, and alkalizers disturb the absorption of both calcium and Vitamin C.

6. Vitamin D is essential for the use of calcium. If you aren't able to expose your body to the sun each day, include a little fish liver oil in your diet.

7. Excessive use of mineral oil laxatives can wash oil-soluble Vitamins A, D, E, and K out of your intestinal tract.

8. If you don't eat whole wheat products, try to add a little wheat germ or wheat germ oil to your diet for additional Vitamin E.

9. Vegetarians should include eggs and milk products in their diet in order to make sure they get all the essential amino acids.

10. If your diet contains fresh, unprocessed foods that are rich in calcium, iron, and iodine, chances are you'll get all the other minerals you need.

5

How to Keep Your Bowels Healthy and Active for Youthful Elimination

If you eat the type of wholesome foods recommended in Chapter 4, you're headed in the right direction as far as your bowels are concerned. But you'll have to observe a special set of rules to assure proper elimination of food waste if you want to be truly youthful and vigorous.

Worry, stress, trips, missed meals, and other disturbing influences will occasionally disturb your bowels enough to temporarily halt the elimination of waste matter. What you do to help yourself can have a great deal to do with how you feel and how you get along with your bowels in time to come.

Everyone suffers from a small amount of constipation at one time or another. This is normal. All you have to do to correct it is to observe the laws of nature. If you fail to do this, or if you try to circumvent nature by using artificial laxatives, you're headed for trouble. Your bowels might even strike back by refusing to function. Any doctor will tell you that most cases of severe, chronic constipation are caused by excessive use of laxatives.

Distension of the lower bowel in unrelieved constipation can cause headache, nervousness, mental confusion, backache, fatigue, and other distressing symptoms. Straining to empty a clogged bowel can cause hernia, hemorrhoids, or anal fissures. Digestion and absorption of nutrients may also be impaired, and this can have far-reaching effects on your general health.

So it's very important to give your bowels the attention they deserve, especially if you want to continue to enjoy the pleasures of healthful eating and youthful health.

THE BIGGEST CAUSE OF CONSTIPATION

The type of food you eat is important in keeping your bowels healthy and active, but food alone is rarely a cause of constipation. Actually, *failure to keep regular toilet appointments is the most common cause of constipation.*

When the food you eat completes its journey through the small intestine, the waste that remains is dumped into the colon or large intestine where it is processed for elimination. Most of the water in the mushy waste is absorbed, so that the waste that remains is made up of a fairly firm solid. When the waste remains in the colon too long, however, too much water is absorbed. This leaves the remaining waste hard, lumpy, and difficult to evacuate, and the longer it stays in the colon the harder it becomes. It may, in fact, become so solidly packed in the rectum that it must sometimes be broken up and removed with a probing finger. The colon itself may become enlarged from overloading, and this can damage important nerves and muscles.

A SEVEN-POINT PLAN TO KEEP YOUR BOWELS MOVING

Most people think of constipation as an "old folk's disease," but it's also common among young people. Consider the case of Janet R., a 28-year-old unmarried secretary.

"I'm just miserable and bloated most of the time," she said the first time she visited my office. "I feel as if I'm carrying around a 20-pound bag of garbage in my abdomen. I can always tell when I need a laxative, because I begin to develop a headache."

When I asked Janet if she went to the toilet every day, she replied "No, only when I take a laxative, which is about every three days."

Here's the seven-point plan I told Janet to follow for two weeks:

1. Drink *two* glasses of fruit or vegetable juice each morning.

2. Eat some raw and dried fruit every day.

3. Eat at the same time every day.

4. Visit the toilet at the same time every day, preferably after each meal.

5. Discontinue the use of all laxatives.

6. Take a warm-water enema every four days if the bowels don't move.

7. Take a little exercise and get a good night's sleep.

After only two weeks on this program, Janet called to say that she was as regular as a schoolgirl. "The plan worked," she said excitedly. "I feel 20 pounds lighter—and I feel great. I have more energy, and I no longer have that sluggish, headachy feeling."

The rest of this chapter will tell you why this plan worked for Janet and how it can work for you. What you learn will be an important part of an overall plan for building youthful health that will give you new zest for living a long and happy life.

How Often Should Your Bowels Move?

There is no set rule that every one can follow in working out a schedule for visiting the toilet. Some people go two or three times a day, while others go only a couple of times a week. The important thing is to *never ignore or resist an urge to visit the toilet.* Remember that feces or waste matter dries very quickly when it is allowed to remain in the lower bowel or rectum. If the urge to defecate is ignored for very long, the bowel will stretch and the urge will vanish. This frequently happens in travelers and other people who "hold back" when toilet facilities are unavailable or not convenient.

An elderly woman who shared a small home with her son and his family became severely constipated because of her reluctance to use the toilet when other members of the family were in the house. Always try to make sure that your house has adequate toilet facilities. Every home should have two toilets—one for "him" and one for "her" whenever possible.

Don't Miss a Toilet Appointment

Try to visit the toilet at the same time every day. Don't let anything else interfere. You can actually train your bowels so that they will empty right on schedule; that is, of course, if you eat regularly and the rest of your day is on schedule.

When you do go to the toilet, be sure to give your bowels plenty of time to move. Try to pick a time when you won't be rushed. Relax. If your muscles are tense and your mind is in a turmoil, the muscular walls of your colon will not push the waste matter down into your rectum where defecation is triggered.

Sitting with your feet on a stool so that your thighs are flexed on your abdomen will aid evacuation of your bowels.

HOW CONSTIPATION CAN CAUSE HEMORRHOIDS AND HERNIA

If your bowels are slow to move, don't try to force them. Straining at the stool is a common cause of hemorrhoids, and it can cause hernia. If you do strain a little occasionally, remember this important rule: *Always exhale when you contract your abdominal muscles.*

When you hold your breath while straining, a build-up of positive pressure in your chest places pressure on the big veins returning to your heart. This causes venous blood to back up into the veins of the rectum. If any of the veins have weak or defective valves, they will become permanently swollen and enlarged. Pressure upon the abdominal organs may also push a loop of intestine right through a weak femoral or inguinal ring in the lower abdomen or groin. Be sure to study the tips on correct breathing in Chapter 7.

If your bowels occasionally fail to move on schedule, don't worry about it. Just be sure to go straight to the toilet when the urge returns, and then continue your regular toilet appointments. Chances are a couple of trips will get you back on schedule.

FORGET ABOUT AUTOINTOXICATION

Don't worry about being "poisoned" by the waste matter that accumulates in your colon when you miss a bowel movement or two. Prolonged or unrelieved constipation can cause considerable discomfort, but no poisoning will occur. Your colon will absorb water from food residue but it will not absorb toxins. If toxins and bacterial by-products do manage to penetrate the walls of the large bowel, they will be filtered from the blood by the liver in its detoxification process.

Once you have determined how many bowel movements are normal for you, whether it's twice a day or twice a week, you'll know when you should take additional steps to aid evacuation of your bowels. If you're accustomed to defecating twice a day, for example, and your bowels are tardy for four or five days, there are a few things you can do to help yourself and your bowels.

FOOD THAT STIMULATE THE BOWELS

All foods stimulate the bowels to some extent, but some are more stimulating than others. Raw fruits and vegetables, for example, aid elimination by contributing bulk-forming cellulose that retains water and "sweeps" the colon. Prunes, figs, raisins, dates, cabbage, beets, salads, apples, and whole grain products are also good laxative foods. One of my patients, a traveling salesman, says that he can always depend upon two tablespoons of fresh beet pulp to move his bowels at the end of a long trip.

Try to eat a couple of servings of fresh fruits and vegetables every day—and eat them raw whenever possible. If your bowels are too sensitive to tolerate the coarse, uncooked cellulose found in some vegetables, it is all right to cook them if you don't boil them to a mush.

Avoid the use of refined and artificial foods whenever possible. In addition to being deficient in the important B vitamins, such foods do not leave enough solid residue to retain water in the lower bowel and to aid bacterial action. The bacteria normally found in your colon are essential for proper digestion and elimination, and their growth is aided by the cellulose found in fruits and vegetables.

If you aren't able to eat properly during the day, you should probably supplement your diet with brewer's yeast and wheat germ for a little additional Vitamin B and roughage.

Go Easy on Bran

A certain amount of bran in the diet will be helpful, but too much can be harmful. There are, in fact, a few people who cannot tolerate pure bran at all, and some of them do better on a smooth diet than on a rough diet. Be careful not to overdo it with "pure bran cereals." Be guided by your experience and by the effect of the foods you eat. Bran does not retain water the way cellulose does. An excessive amount may clog your colon with a dry, tightly packed residue, or it might cause diarrhea.

Bulk Without Roughage

If you must reduce the amount of roughage in your diet for some reason, or if fresh fruits and vegetables are not available, you can supply your intestinal tract with a non-irritating bulk by eating supplements made from agar-agar or from psyllium seed. A gelatinous-like extract from either of these two products will pass through your intestines without being digested, and it will retain water to provide bulk without irritating the stomach or the colon.

HOW TO CULTIVATE FRIENDLY BACTERIA IN YOUR BOWELS

Did you know that about 80 percent of the material evacuated by the normal, healthy bowel is composed of bacteria? Many of these bacteria are of a type called lactobacillus—or should be. When they are present in the bowel in sufficient numbers, they prevent putrefaction and destroy hostile, gas-forming bacteria by producing lactic acid. They also help to prevent constipation by keeping the environment of the bowel normal.

Excessive gas that has a foul odor means that putrefactive bacteria are feeding on undigested food. This may mean that you do not have enough lactobacillus in your colon.

You can increase the number of friendly bacteria in your intestinal tract by eating cultured yogurt or by drinking acidophilus milk. Since lactobacillus must feed upon milk sugar to multiply, you should also include a little whey, milk, powdered milk or some other milk product containing lactose or milk sugar. Once the bacteria have been planted in your colon, they will continue to multiply if your diet contains milk sugar. Whey, which is about 70 percent lactose, is commonly taken along with acidophilus culture. Both of these products are available in health food stores.

The spores of lactobacillus are unaffected by stomach acid, and go directly to the colon where they produce an acid that kills disease-producing germs. Lactose also passes through the intestinal tract unchanged until it gets to the colon where it may be absorbed or serve as food for lactobacillus.

Large amounts of lactose in the diet, especially in the form of buttermilk or acidophilus milk, will ferment and form organic acids that prevent putrefaction. An excessive amount of milk sugar can form an uncomfortable amount of gas, but it is harmless and does not have the foul odor produced by putrefaction of protein.

BEWARE OF LAXATIVES!

With a little time and patience, simple constipation can be corrected with regular toilet appointments and an increased intake of fruits and vegetables. Even if your bowels don't move for a few days, no harm will result. If you become impatient and take a laxative to forcefully move your bowels, you may upset your entire intestinal tract.

Actually, the only portion of the intestinal tract that really needs to be cleaned out when you are constipated is the rectum, or the last eight inches of the colon. It is here that dry, impacted waste matter accumulates to clog the bowel. This "plug" can usually be removed with a simple enema.

When you take a laxative, you upset 25 feet of intestine. If you take laxatives regularly, your entire intestinal tract will soon fail to respond to the stimulation of ordinary food. In other words, you eventually become dependent upon the use of laxatives.

Most persons who take a laxative when they miss a bowel movement or two do not realize that they are purging their small and large intestines. When they fail to have another bowel movement after three or four days, they take another laxative, believing they are still constipated. Actually, it may take several days for enough waste matter to accumulate in the rectum to create an urge to defecate.

It wouldn't take more than a few weeks of such improper use of laxatives to do the body great harm. If the laxatives are taken too often, the bowels will be emptied prematurely. This can deprive the body of youth-building nutrients by forcing the intestinal tract to eliminate partially digested food.

Self-Induced Diarrhea

Many people who take laxatives are not constipated and do not need them. Arthur C., for example, took laxatives frequently. "I just cannot gain any weight," he complained, "and I'm tired all the time." When I asked him about the shape of his stools, he said that his stools didn't have any shape, that they were soft and mushy. "But that's better than being constipated," he added.

Actually, Arthur was suffering from self-induced diarrhea. Excessive loss of water and undigested food was depriving his body of nourishment. All he had to do to "break the laxative habit" was to quit taking laxatives. Once he understood that it wasn't absolutely necessary to have a bowel movement every day, he got along fine—and he felt better.

Breaking the Laxative Habit

If you suffer from chronic constipation that is characterized by hard, dry stools, and your bowels are truly addicted to laxative stimulation, you may have to withdraw gradually from the use of laxatives while increasing your intake of fruits, vegetables, and juices. Cascara sagrada, a mild bark laxative, can replace more powerful laxatives until withdrawal is complete. After a few weeks, you should eliminate laxatives altogether and let nature take its course. It shouldn't be too long before your bowels begin to move normally again.

If you are an elderly person and you think that the muscles and nerves controlling your bowels are too weak to do the job alone, ask your doctor about the continued use of a mild laxative. But be sure not to use it so often that your stools are soft and mushy rather than moist and firm.

Don't Use Mineral Oils

You should never use mineral oil as a laxative; it will absorb the fat soluble vitamins and then eliminate them through your bowels. The oil may also leak from your rectum during the day, causing considerable discomfort or embarrassment. If you should accidently inhale a few drops of the oil, a serious form of pneumonia could develop.

You can, however, safely inject three ounces of mineral oil into your rectum just before retiring at night in order to soften the feces for a morning evacuation or an enema.

HOW TO TAKE AN ENEMA

If you do become constipated occasionally, and your bowels do not move for four or five days, a simple enema may be all you'll need to gain relief. Take it during one of your regular toilet appointments so that you'll be able to get back on schedule.

Mix one teaspoonful of table salt into one pint of warm water, or two teaspoons into a quart. You don't need all the stuff that some people mix into enema water. Soap suds, for example, can irritate your colon and cause pain and spasm.

Lubricate the enema tip with KY Jelly, Vaseline, or baby oil and then insert it two to four inches into the rectum. The container holding the water should be suspended 12 to 18 inches above the buttocks so that the water will flow into the rectum when the tube is unclamped. Let the water flow slowly—by manipulating the clamp—over a period of several minutes so that it won't be expelled prematurely by cramps.

If possible, the water should be retained in the rectum for five to ten minutes so that there'll ample time for the feces to soften.

The enema may be taken while lying on one side with the uppermost thigh and leg flexed or while in a knee-chest position with the body supported by the forearms and the knees. The latter position is probably best for retaining a full quart of water.

The Dangers of Colonics

Except in special cases, I do not recommend the use of "high colonics" in which the entire colon is irrigated. It's now well known that the large colon completes work left undone by the small intestine. If the colon is repeatedly flooded with water that flows in and out under pressure, a loss of important bacteria and their secretions may allow the growth of hostile and putrefactive organisms. The mucous membrane lining the walls of the colon may also be washed away, leaving the colon inflamed, irritable, and spastic. This can lead to either diarrhea or constipation.

EXERCISE AND SLEEP

Any kind of exercise will aid bowel movements by relaxing nerves and stimulating the circulation. Simple sit-ups will do wonders by toning the abdominal muscles and massaging the intestinal tract. Try to do a few sit-ups each evening after work, or a few hours before supper. Well-developed abdominal muscles will provide your body with a youthful, natural corset.

Since unrelieved nervous tension can deprive the bowels of the nerve impulses they need to function smoothly, you should make sure that you get a good night's sleep each night. This will speed digestion of the food you've eaten during the day so that your bowels will be ready to empty in the morning. Chapter 14 will explain clearly and simply how you can get the most out of your sleep.

DRINK PLENTY OF LIQUIDS

If you drink plenty of water and eat a variety of fruits and vegetables that contain cellulose, your stools will be moist, firm, and well formed—if you keep regular toilet appointments.

Fruit juices are a good source of water, and they contain organic acids that stimulate the intestinal tract. This is why so many people take lemon juice in warm water each morning before breakfast.

Coffee is a powerful intestinal stimulate, but it can have harmful effects by lowering blood sugar; it can also constrict blood vessels and overstimulate the nervous system. If you do drink coffee, drink it just before your regular toilet appointment in the morning or at noon—never just before bedtime.

ANOTHER WARNING ABOUT ANTACIDS

Several times throughout this book, you have been warned about possible losses of vitamins and minerals from the use of antacids and alkalizers. Actually, the hydrochloric acid secreted by your stomach is so important in the digestion of food that you should *never* take an alkalizer unless your doctor tells you that your stomach is secreting too much acid.

Medical scientists have recently discovered that a *deficiency* of hydrochloric acid in the stomach can cause digestive disturbances that are similar to those caused by too much acid. So why risk anemia, vitamin deficiency, soft bones, intestinal flatulence, and other disorders by using guesswork in treating yourself with alkalizers. There are many people who have stomachs that do not secrete enough acid to properly digest the food they eat. They certainly shouldn't take alkalizers when they overeat.

PAIN MEANS DANGER

If constipation occurs with pain, fever, cramps, and other symptoms, or is alternated with diarrhea, you may be suffering from something more serious than a clogged rectum. An intestinal obstruction, for example, can cause abdominal pain that may be accompanied by vomiting and fever.

In some cases of spastic constipation, in which abdominal pains, excessive gas, and inflammation of the colon are associated with alternating diarrhea and constipation, medical attention and a special soft diet may be necessary.

Remember that simple constipation is rarely associated with abdominal pain. *Don't ever take a laxative to move your bowels in an effort to relieve pain.* An inflamed or swollen appendix, which is very often accompanied by pain and constipation, could be ruptured by laxatives that cause abdominal cramping.

Chronic diarrhea also warrants medical attention. If it continues unrelieved, it can literally drain your body of water and nutrients. There are many disorders of the colon and rectum, such as colitis, tumors, diverticulitis, and so on, that can cause diarrhea, and many of them must be diagnosed by X-ray examination.

SUMMARY

1. Include plenty of fresh fruits and vegetables, whole grain products, and fruit juices in your daily diet for intestinal stimulation as well as for youth-building vitamins and minerals.

2. Set up a regular schedule for visiting the toilet and stick with it, but never resist an urge to empty your bowels at any time.

3. Remember that it's perfectly normal for some people to have a bowel movement only two or three times a week.

4. If nervous tension or an interruption in your daily habits results in failure to have an expected bowel movement, don't worry about it. Chances are your bowels will move during your next visit to the toilet—if not before then.

5. If your bowels fail to move adequately for several days and your stool becomes hard and dry, a simple warm-water enema may get you back on schedule.

6. Since only the rectum, or the lower portion of the colon, is usually involved in simple constipation, it's rarely necessary to irrigate the entire colon with "high colonics."

7. If you must eliminate roughage in your diet for some reason, you can get non-irritating bulk from agar-agar or psyllium seed extract.

8. Cultured yogurt or acidophilus milk with whey or milk sugar will aid digestion and elimination by increasing the number of lactobacillus acidophilus in your colon.

9. Remember that if you do take a laxative it may be several days before enough waste matter will accumulate in your lower colon or rectum to create an urge to visit the toilet.

10. Whenever failure to have a bowel movement is accompanied by pain, cramps, nausea, or other symptoms of illness, don't take a laxative. Let your doctor recommend treatment.

6

How to Combat the Aging Process with Improved Circulation of Blood

There is an old adage that says that man is as old as his arteries. Since every cell in the body depends upon the circulation of blood for oxygen, nutrients, hormones, and waste disposal, it's not hard to understand that when the circulation begins to fail the body begins to die. Research has revealed that the amount of blood circulating through the muscle tissue of the average old person decreases as much as 40 percent.

Chapter 8 will tell you how to enrich your blood with the iron it needs to supply your tissues with oxygen. And Chapter 9 will tell you how to alter your diet to prevent hardening of your arteries. In this chapter, you'll learn how to *improve* your circulation so that every portion of your body will receive a generous supply of nourishing blood. You don't have to be "old" to benefit from these instructions. In fact, the younger you are when you begin to make an effort to improve your circulation, the better your chances of staying young.

BREATHING FOR BETTER CIRCULATION

The first thing you should do to improve your circulation of blood is to observe one simple breathing rule. And here it is: *Take a deep breath several times a day, expanding your rib cage as much as you can.* You'll learn more about the effects of breathing in Chapter 7.

HELP YOUR VEINS BY REVERSING THE PULL OF GRAVITY

Of course, you can't really reverse the pull of gravity, but you can reverse the effect that gravity has on the veins of your body. You know that blood leaves the heart through arteries and then returns through veins. Since most of the veins of the body are below the heart, the pull of gravity greatly interferes with the circulation of blood when you stand erect, especially when you are standing still. In fact, when you stand for 30 minutes or longer, the volume of blood circulating through your body may decrease as much as 15 percent because of a seepage of blood fluids into tissue spaces. This is why some people complain of swollen ankles after sitting or standing all day.

Whenever possible, *elevate your legs so that venous blood can flow "down hill," and so that excess fluid will be drained out of your feet and legs.* Just lie down on the floor and prop your feet up on a chair, or lie down on a slant board with your feet anchored at the high end of the board. I know some office workers who use a slant board during their coffee breaks. All of them report that in addition to aiding their circulation, the upside down position on the board relieves fatigue and improves thinking. It can also relieve backache by stretching the spine to relieve pressure on joints and discs.

Caution: If you have heart trouble or high blood pressure, don't elevate the end of your slant board more than 12 inches. Return to a sitting position when you begin to feel uncomfortable.

A FLAT ABDOMEN IS IMPORTANT FOR GOOD CIRCULATION

Everyone knows that a bulging, oversized waistline is fatiguing and unsightly, but few people know that it can have a damaging effect on the circulation or blood. When the abdominal muscles sag, certain important veins also sag. Abdominal organs become sluggish and congested with stagnant blood. You obviously cannot allow this to happen if you want to live a long, youthful life.

How Your Muscles Support Your Veins

Arteries have thick and elastic walls that expand with each heart beat and then recoil between beats to act as a subsidiary pump. Veins, however, have thin, weak walls. Without the support of the surrounding tissues, your veins would stretch and sag lifelessly under the weight of the blood they contain.

In the arms and legs, where veins weave around and through the muscles, blood flow is stimulated by simple muscular contraction. In the abdomen, however, where huge veins drain blood from the lower body as well as from important organs, the veins are supported by the abdominal walls so that venous blood flow may be aided by the pumping action of the diaphragm. When your waistline "goes to pot," all of the abdominal veins are pulled down and squeezed by displaced organs. Capillary beds, which consist of tiny vessels that connect veins and arteries, become so enlarged that the volume of blood circulating through your body is greatly reduced.

The Importance of Sit-Ups

You don't have to let your abdomen become a stagnant pool of venous blood. *A half-dozen bent-knee sit-ups each day would be enough to keep your abdominal muscles tight and elastic.* (See Figure 6-1.)

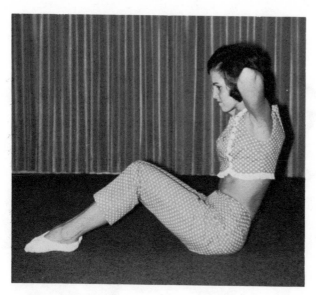

Figure 6-1. *The knees should always be kept bent during sit-ups.*

If you find sit-ups too difficult to do, you can do *trunk curls,* in which you curl only your head and shoulders up from the floor, as in beginning a sit-up. Performing this exercise on a slant board will further aid circulation by allowing venous blood to drain out of your legs and lower abdomen. Anchor your feet at the high end of the board, place your hands behind your head, and do 12 to 15 trunk curls. (See Figure 6-2.)

It's important to keep your lower back on the board and curl only your head and shoulders up from the board in order to activate your abdominal muscles.

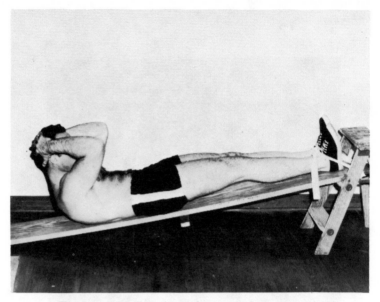

Figure 6-2. *Trunk curls on a slant board aid circulation and activate the abdominal muscles.*

A Case History of Trunk Curls on a Slant Board

Susan G., a thirty-year-old practical nurse who complained of abdominal pains, constipation, and swollen ankles, eliminated *all* of these complaints by doing 15 trunk curls on a slant board each day after leaving the hospital where she worked.

"I'm really glad to get rid of all those aches and pains," she said after doing the exercises for several weeks, "but I'm even more pleased to get rid of that stomach. I no longer have to wear a girdle, and my husband says I look ten years younger! I know I sure feel better."

Why not put a slant board in your bedroom or in your office and do a few trunk curls after work or just before supper? The improvement in circulation from just a few seconds of effort will add years to your life. You may also regain some of the physical vigor that you thought had been lost forever.

TRY WALKING!

Because of the importance of the muscles in supporting and massaging the veins of the legs, you should try to walk a couple of blocks each day. The contraction of the large muscles in the calves and thighs will pump blood through the legs by alternately squeezing and releasing veins and capillaries.

Walking can be entertaining as well as healthful. When did you last walk along a country road or through the woods for a closer look at the world of nature? Don't get so involved in the ways of the city that you forget how to walk solely for the pleasure of walking.

Breathe deeply while you walk. And don't forget to expand your rib cage occasionally so that thoracic suction will pull venous blood toward your heart.

Walking will also raise the body temperature slightly, and it will decrease the viscosity of blood so that it will flow more easily through small veins and capillaries.

USING A ROCKING CHAIR TO HELP YOUR HEART

If you don't like to walk, or if you aren't able to walk for some reason, you can aid the circulation of blood with a rocking chair. A brisk rocking motion will activate the muscles of the body in a pumping action that will actually aid the heart in pumping blood. Old people who are not very active and who spend much of their time sitting should always sit in a rocking chair rather than a stationary chair.

IMPROVING LYMPH FLOW WITH MASSAGE

Simple exercise is best for increasing the flow of blood

through the body, since the oxygen debt created by exercise will also stimulate heart rate and respiration. But if you would like to flush out your muscles without making any effort at all, you can have someone give you a body massage. Manual compression of the muscles will empty lymph channels as well as veins so that a fresh flow of blood and lymph can remove toxins and wastes that cause premature aging. Stimulation of nerve fibers by rubbing the skin will also improve the function of the liver, kidneys, and other organs.

Technique of Massage

Apply a small amount of lubricant to the skin and stroke or knead the muscles. Always *rub toward the heart* so that you will follow the direction of the venous blood flow. Just cup one or both hands over a muscle and apply firm overlapping strokes until the entire length of the muscle or limb is covered.

It isn't necessary to hack or pound a muscle. A slow, gentle stroking massage will relax muscles as well as stimulate the circulation.

Mineral oil is a good massage lubricant. Cocoa butter is best for hairy skin. Most masseurs prefer to mix a little mineral oil in alcohol. The alcohol evaporates quickly, leaving a small amount of oil evenly distributed over the skin.

Follow the massage with a warm shower that is gradually turned down to a comfortably cool temperature.

If you don't suffer from dry skin (see Chapter 12), an alcohol rub following the massage will stimulate circulation as well as remove the oil.

HOW TO STIMULATE BLOOD FLOW WITH WATER

Applying water to the skin is probably the easiest and most effective way to increase circulation throughout the body. The blood vessels in the skin, for example, can hold about one-quarter of the total amount of blood in the body.

When blood is drawn to the skin by hot water and then driven inward by cold water, the entire vascular system is given a good workout. Also, the stimulation of nerve fibers in the skin reaches deep into the organs of the body.

Properly applied, cold water is a potent metabolic and circulatory tonic that will keep your body young and vigorous.

Hot water will increase circulation when applied to an isolated area of the body, but it has a depressing effect on the nerves and muscles. Cold water, however, when applied over the entire body, will increase your working ability about 30 percent. This tonic effect on muscles, nerves, blood vessels, and organs helps to postpone the aging process by speeding repair and regeneration of body tissue.

A Simple Bath Tonic

The reaction of the body to cold water is much more effective if it is preceded by a hot bath. Soaking in a tub of hot water for about five minutes, for example, will increase circulation in the skin by dilating blood vessels. If the bath is continued for several minutes, a maximum amount of blood will flow near the surface of the skin in an effort to cool the body. Then, when you step under a cool shower, constriction of the blood vessels in the skin will drive the blood into the muscles. (Most persons will prefer to begin with a warm shower and then gradually turn it down to cold.)

About one minute of exposure to cold water is long enough for a good reaction. Too long an exposure to water colder than 60 degrees can be fatiguing, and it may lower your resistance to infection.

For cold water treatment to be beneficial in building youthful health and vigor, it must be followed by a sensation of warmth and exhilaration. If you suffer a chill, or if your skin turns blue rather than pink following immersion in cold water, your vascular system is not adapting to the sudden change in temperature. Try to avoid water that is cold enough to give you a chill.

Even if you are perfectly healthy, extremely hot or cold water can paralyze or "switch off" the nerve reflexes that regulate the flow of blood through the skin. So don't join a winter swim club or torture yourself with unbearably hot "spring water."

> **Caution**: The older a person is, the more sluggish his circulatory reaction may be to cold water. If you're over 60 and you chill easily, or if you have high blood pressure or heart trouble, don't bathe in very hot or very cold water. Just take a warm shower and then gradually turn it down to a comfortably cool temperature.

The Cold Towel Rub for the Verve of Youth

If your vascular system reacts beneficially to cold water, and you would like to systematically stimulate every portion of your body, you can try a cold towel rub. Have someone apply the treatment for you if possible.

Fill two pails with cold water—about 60 degrees Fahrenheit. Put a couple of ice cubes in the water to make sure that it stays cold. Soak a large linen towel in each pail.

Wring out the towel in the first pail and apply it to one arm. The entire arm should be rubbed with the towel until the towel becomes slightly warm. Then return the towel to the first pail and wring out the second towel for the other arm.

Treatment of the arms, legs, back, chest, and abdomen should not take longer than five minutes, Each part of the body should be dried and covered before going to the next.

After the treatment is completed, you should feel warm and stimulated. The effect of the cold moisture and massage on the nervous system and the circulation will charge you with the verve of youth.

The Cold Mitten Rub for Quick Energy

If you don't have a partner who can give you a cold towel massage, you can do it yourself by rubbing your body with thick towel-type mittens that have been dipped in ice water.

Place the mittens and a pail of cold water alongside your bath tub so that you can rub your body immediately following a hot bath. Just remain sitting in the tub after draining the water and then slip on the mittens and place the pail between your legs. Go over your entire body as rapidly as possible. When the rub is completed, you should feel a surge of energy that will literally spring you out of the tub.

A service station operator I know who attends night school takes a cold mitten rub each night before beginning classes. "It does wonders for me," he said. "It really wakes me up—and I can think more clearly. My wife says that I have more energy than our 18-year-old son. But I don't believe I could make it without rubbing myself with cold water."

A store manager who finishes each day feeling "tired and sluggish" restores his energy each night by taking a hot bath and a cold mitten rub just as soon as he gets home. "The bath and the rub certainly make me feel better," he told me in my office one day. "I enjoy my evenings much more than I did before I started the water treatment. I never used to feel like going bowling or taking in a movie."

The effects of the water and the massage simply stimulated the physiological processes in these two men so that they experienced a rejuvenation of youthful ambition and ability. You can get the same results. Anything you can do to make you *feel* younger will help you combat the aging process. When you feel young, you *think* young, and the power of the mind can work wonders.

TRY A SITZ BATH FOR A SEXUAL AWAKENING

If you feel that your sexual powers are waning and you

would like to try circulatory stimulation to regain some of your former capacity, you should include a contrast sitz bath in your water-treatment routine.

A 65-year-old retired navy chief who had complained of sexual impotency found that the bath was so effective that he suddenly decided to get married. It's only fair to mention, however, that he had also been drinking sarsaparilla tea and eating pumpkin seeds, both of which contain substances that are believed to stimulate male hormones.

Circulatory stimulation of the pelvic area is important for many reasons other than sexual rejuvenation. The effect of contrasting water temperature on the pelvic nerves, for example, is great for relieving constipation caused by a "lazy" or atonic colon. Hemorrhoids may also be relieved.

Sitz Bath Technique

Fill one wash tub with hot water (about 110 degrees F.) and another with cold water (about 45 degrees F.). Sit down in the hot water for about five minutes and then in the cold water for about five minutes. Repeat the hot-to-cold cycle at least twice.

The tremendous circulatory stimulation of such treatment will flush out vessels and glands and awaken their function.

HOW TO CLEANSE YOUR BLOOD WITH A LIVER PACK

The liver is the largest organ in the body. It services the blood by filtering out toxins and keeping the blood stream supplied with blood cells, protein, sugar (glucose), and other important body-building and blood-building elements. So it might be a good idea to stimulate the circulation of blood through the liver by applying a "liver pack."

In addition to aiding the passage of waste-loaded venous blood through the liver, the application of moist heat will dilate tiny arteries and capillaries so that the liver itself will receive an increased supply of fresh arterial blood.

The liver is such an important organ that when circulation through it is slowed by congestion or clogged vessels, your whole body suffers. Toxins accumulate in your blood to cause aging sluggishness and fatigue.

Liver Pack Technique

Fold a piece of toweling or calico six or eight times and wring it out in hot water that contains a little mustard or oil of wintergreen.

Place the pack over the liver (just beneath the ribs on the right side of the abdomen) and cover it with a sheet of rubber or plastic. You can keep the pack hot for about 20 minutes by applying a hot water bottle or by illuminating it with the rays of an infrared lamp.

Caution: Use only a small amount of mustard or oil of wintergreen to begin with, lest you blister your skin. Try mixing a tablespoonful of mustard into a large pan of water. You can determine from experience how much to use to give your skin a comfortably red glow. Remove the pack if pain or discomfort occurs.

Important: When you remove the pack, sponge the heated area with cold water for maximum stimulation of blood flow.

THE NEW HYDROVASCULAR EXERCISES
FOR A YOUTHFUL BODY

If you're fortunate enough to live near the seashore, you can take special "salt-water exercises" that will stimulate your circulation, improve your physical appearance, and build up your endurance. Fresh air, sunshine, and salt water, when combined with active contraction of the muscles, add up to the most potent metabolic and circulatory tonic that nature has to offer. Unlike the calisthenics that you have already tried and given up, *the new revolutionary hydro-vascular exercises are fun and refreshing.*

Special Anti-Gravity Effect

Exercising in salt water has one important effect that cannot be duplicated on dry land. Because of the high salt and mineral content of sea water, the pressure of the water against the lower portion of the body will greatly reduce the hydrostatic pressure of the blood in the veins of the legs and the abdomen. In other words, the weight of the blood and the size of the veins will be greatly reduced in the weightless environment, thus aiding the flow of blood in overcoming the pull of gravity.

If you suffer from varicose veins, the support offered by the pressure of the water should enable you to exercise without increasing distension in swollen veins. In fact, hydro-vascular exercises should *reduce* venous congestion in your legs. Hemorrhoids would also benefit.

If there isn't any salt water in your area, you can do the exercises in a lake or a pool—or in any body of water. Fresh water is not quite as buoyant as salt water, but it will have nearly the same effect on the circulation of blood.

Water Temperature

Outdoor water exercise should be taken only on warm days, preferably during the summer, and the water should not be any colder than 60 degrees. An ideal temperature would be 65 to 68 degrees.

Since the temperature of the skin is normally about 93 degrees, any water temperature below 80 degrees will feel cold. An air temperature of 75 degrees may feel comfortable, but water with the same temperature may feel very cold to some people. Water always feels colder than air of the same temperature, so don't try to compare the two for bathing purposes. The water should, of course, be cold enough to cause a circulatory reaction, but almost any outdoor body of water will be cold enough for the average person.

Try to take advantage of the summer months to expose your body to sun, air, and water. *The sea, or a backyard pond, can be your fountain of youth.*

The Experience of a Beach Couple

A 44-year-old motel operator and his wife who live on a Florida beach spend about ten minutes each day exercising in the Gulf of Mexico. They do the same hydrovascular exercises that I am about to recommend for you.

"I used to be thin and bony," the wife said, "but the water exercises have filled out my body quite nicely. I no longer suffer from constipation, leg cramps, and insomnia. My friends say I look younger now than I did ten years ago. I certainly *feel* younger. My husband has even taken a new interest in me."

The husband was also trim and fit, and he reported that the varicose veins in his legs no longer bothered him. "We try to do the exercises together," he said, " and we really feel good after doing them. The water is very stimulating. We actually enjoy doing the exercises—if you can call it exercising."

There is something about the air of a seashore that makes you *want* to exercise. And when your skin is bathed with cool water, your energy doubles and triples. If you don't like to exercise in public or in a stuffy room, try the new hydrovascular exercises. Do them at least twice a week for best results. If you have access to an indoor pool, you can do them throughout the year for a truly youthful body.

Caution: The colder the water the greater the stimulation. If the water is colder than 65 degrees, however, it wouldn't be a good idea to stay in longer than four or five minutes. Stop the exercises when you begin to feel mildly fatigued. For safety reasons, always try to have a friend or partner present when you go into the water. If the air is cool when you leave the water, dry your skin immediately.

Six Hydrovascular Exercises to Promote Youthfulness

Stand erect in water that's about shoulder deep when you do these exercises.

1. Walk through the water as fast as you can. The resistance of the water will give your leg muscles (and your heart and lungs) a real workout. Lean forward a little so that you can build momentum.

2. Stand on one straight leg and swing the opposite straight leg forward and backward with a rapid count. Several repetitions with each leg will exercise thigh, abdominal, and back muscles. (See Figure 6-3.)

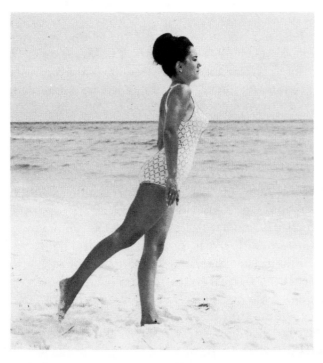

Figure 6-3. *Hydrovascular exercise No. 2.*

3. Hold your arms out straight at shoulder level (under water) and sweep them forward and backward. Keep your fingers together and your hands open so that water resistance will be increased. The faster you move your arms, the greater the resistance of the water. (See Figure 6-4.)

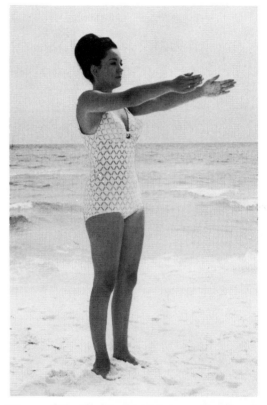

Figure 6-4. *Hydrovascular exercise No. 3.*

This is an excellent exercise for chest and back muscles, for women as well as for men. Do as many repetitions as necessary to produce mild fatigue.

4. Stand on one leg and lift the knee of the opposite leg as high as you can. Let the knee bend freely so that you can lift your thigh as close to your abdomen as possible. Exercise both legs equally. This hip-flexion exercise will tone muscles as well as pump blood. (See Figure 6-5.)

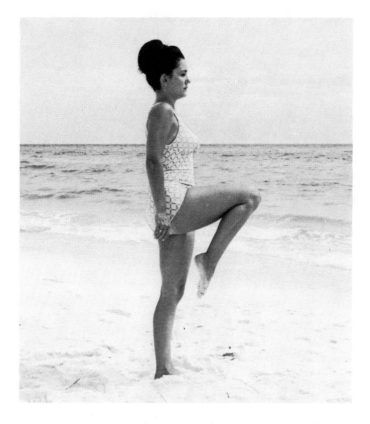

Figure 6-5. *Hydrovascular exercise No. 4.*

5. Stand erect with your feet about 12 inches apart, both hands on your hips, and your elbows flared out on each side. Keep your arms braced and rigid so that they won't move; then rotate your body on its vertical axis (in a

standing twist), first to one side and then to the other in continuous movement. The resistance of your arms moving through the water will give your torso a good workout. Rotate your body just fast enough to produce comfortable fatigue in 15 to 20 repetitions.

This is a fine exercise for trimming the abdomen and firming the hips. Do it as often as you can if you are overweight.

6. After completing the first five exercises, you should be breathing rather heavily. This final exercise will aid breathing as well as circulation. (See Figure 6-6.)

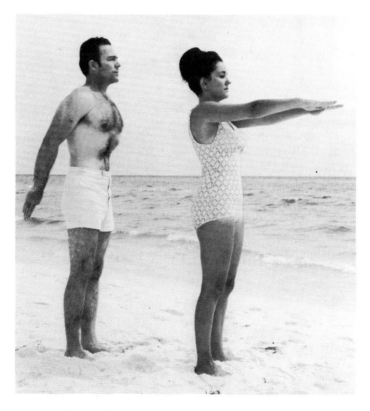

Figure 6-6. *Hydrovascular exercise No. 6.*

Extend your arms out straight in front with both palms flat and facing downward. Keep your arms locked out straight and sweep them down in front and alongside your body. Inhale deeply as your arms go down. Exhale as you return your arms to starting position.

HOW TO MAKE "SEA WATER" FOR YOUR TUB BATH

If you can't go to the seashore, you might want to occasionally fill your bath tub with "home-made" sea water.

For a simple salt bath, you can add three to five pounds of common table salt to a tub of water. For "sea water," however, you should mix seven pounds of sodium chloride (salt), one pound magnesium chloride, and one-half pound of magnesium sulfate in 30 gallons of cool water. The high mineral and salt content of such water is highly stimulating to the skin. Follow the bath with a cool shower.

FOR THE ROBUST: A HOT SHOWER AND A COLD PLUNGE

If you're not elderly and you don't have heart disease or high blood pressure, you might want to try following a hot shower with a cold plunge for a really vigorous tonic. For this to be beneficial, however, the cold plunge should immediately follow the hot shower. You should *never* stand around in drafts of cool air after leaving a hot shower.

If you have access to an indoor swimming pool, take a brief but fairly hot shower before jumping into the water. If it doesn't prove to be refreshing and invigorating, don't try it again.

When I was in the navy, I used to swim in a cold water pool that had hot and cold showers just a few feet away from the pool. On days when the water seemed a little colder than usual, I discovered that if I stood under a hot shower for a few minutes before diving into the pool I could withstand the shock of the water much better. And after a brief, vigorous swim, I left the water feeling tremendously energetic.

Caution: You should *never* take a cold plunge following exercise that has made you perspire. When your body temperature has been raised by exercising, and your muscles are congested with blood, your circulatory system cannot adapt to a sudden change in temperature as it does when only the skin has been warmed. Whether you are perspiring from hot weather or from exercise, always "cool off" by getting under a warm shower and then gradually turning it down to cold.

A similar warning can be sounded about exposure to intense heat. If you take sauna baths or steam baths, take them after a cooling shower, never after "working up a sweat."

"Sponging" Your Tissues with Water

If you swim only occasionally, remember that it is not a good idea to jump into cold water when your skin has been chilled. The circulation in the skin may be paralyzed by the shock, so that you leave the water chilled to the bone, shivering, and covered with "goose bumps." When the skin has been heated, however, an increased amount of blood circulating through the skin will provide a vascular cushion that will *prevent* shock. In fact, a plunge into cool water should be a pleasant contrast.

Exposing warmed skin to cold water will drive the blood inward by constricting the blood vessels in the skin. But when you leave the water after a brief swim, the secondary reaction will bring the blood back to the skin, giving you a warm, pleasant glow.

The large amount of blood involved in this physiological "sponging" of the tissues will open tiny vascular channels and contribute to the formation of firm, youthful tissue.

SUMMARY

1. Cold water properly applied to the skin is a very

effective circulatory and metabolic tonic.

2. A hot bath followed by a cool shower (gradually turned down to cold) will "exercise" the vascular system by drawing blood to the skin and then driving it back into the muscles.

3. Contraction and relaxation of the muscles during walking will aid circulation by pushing blood through the veins of the legs.

4. Rocking in a rocking chair will aid circulation in elderly persons who do not get much exercise.

5. Try to elevate your legs several times a day, or lie on a slant board with your head down and your feet up, so that lymph will be drained out of tissue spaces in your feet and legs.

6. Keep your abdomen flat by doing bent-knee sit-ups (or trunk curls) so that veins and organs in your abdomen will be supported by a natural, muscular corset.

7. Extreme or sudden changes in water temperature should be avoided by old people or persons suffering from high blood pressure or heart disease.

8. Towels wrung out in water that has been spiked with mustard or oil of wintergreen can be placed over the liver to stimulate circulation of blood and removal of toxins.

9. An alternate hot and cold sitz bath (limited to the pelvic area) will increase circulation to sexual organs and improve bowel function.

10. Exercising while standing in water will relieve pressure in veins as well as aid venous circulation in overcoming the pull of gravity.

7

How to Breathe Away Poisons and Tone Your Body with Oxygen for Youthful Energy

Before you learn the secret of enriching your blood with oxygen-carrying iron, there are a few simple breathing rules that you should observe to make sure that you keep your red blood cells supplied with oxygen. Each time your heart beats, venous blood is pumped through the lungs for a fresh supply of oxygen. But if all of the air sacs of both lungs are not filled with clean, fresh air, your blood may not pick up adequate oxygen, and it may not unload its waste products. Consequently, your whole program for youthfulness will be penalized.

Unfortunately, most people are "shallow breathers," which means that they rarely breathe deeply enough to fully aerate the far corners of their lungs. As a result, carbon dioxide and stale air accumulate to prevent the exchange of carbon dioxide for oxygen.

Tissue cells must have oxygen to feed the chemical processes of life and to neutralize waste products. Without adequate oxygen, body tissue breaks down, waste clogs cells and capillaries, and the brain does not function efficiently. A backing up of carbon dioxide in the body causes a progressive deterioration of both mind and body.

HOW THE AGING PROCESS CAN BE CHECKED

Oscar C., a retired boiler maker who spent most of his time sitting around the house, was becoming increasingly "weak, irritable, and forgetful." His wife and children all remarked that he seemed to be growing old very fast since his retirement. When they asked me for advice, I suggested that he take up some type of physical activity that would get him outdoors—something that would stimulate his heart rate and respiration. He began doing yard work. When I saw him again a few months later, he was hard at work painting and repairing his home. He was obviously happy, energetic, and mentally alert. The deep breathing and the circulatory stimulation that resulted from the work he was doing had simply increased the flow of oxygen-rich blood to his mind, his body, and his muscles. The aging process, in this case, had actually been reversed to some extent.

If you combine what you learn in this chapter with what you learn in other chapters of this book, you can *delay* the aging process by doing nothing more than making a few simple changes in your day-to-day living habits.

"CHEST BREATHING" INCREASES THE CIRCULATION OF BLOOD

Just about everyone knows that we breathe to exchange carbon dioxide for oxygen. But what most people don't know is that breathing also aids the circulation of blood. In fact, without the assistance provided by the act of breathing, the heart would quickly break down from overwork. So how you breathe can be important. You can actually breathe a certain way to *increase* the amount of blood flowing through your body.

There are, of course, many factors that aid the circulation of blood. Each time the heart beats, for example, the arteries expand to accommodate the outpouring of blood. Then, between beats, the recoil of the elastic arteries keeps the blood circulating until it reaches the veins. Muscular contraction helps move blood through the arms and legs by squeezing and releasing the veins so that they are alternately filled with and emptied of blood. When venous blood reaches the large thoracic and abdominal veins, however, it can barely overcome the pull of gravity in its uphill journey to the heart. This is where respiration offers assistance.

The pressure of the blood in the arteries is normally about 130 millimeters of mercury when it first leaves the heart. But by the time it completes its circuit through the body and returns to the heart, the pressure has dropped to about 5 millimeters of water. Each time you inhale, however, the same negative pressure that draws air into your lungs also exerts a suction effect on the big veins in your chest. In addition to this, your diaphragm moves downward to compress the veins in your abdomen. The combined action of your thorax and your diaphragm acts as a subsidiary pump that actually pulls and pushes venous blood back to your heart. This raises the venous pressure in your chest from nearly zero to about 85 millimeters of water, which is quite a boost for your circulation.

Breathe deeply when you're breathless from exertion or groggy from desk work. When you feel that you need a little extra oxygen or that your circulation is sluggish, *expand your chest when you take a deep breath.* Breathe up into the top of your lungs. This will increase the flow of blood through your lungs and speed the transportation of oxygen to your tissues. Waste products and debris that interfere with the "respiration" of tissue cells will be washed away by rivers of fresh blood. Worn tissue cells will be quickly repaired or replaced, keeping your tissues young and firm.

Breath Holding Can Be Dangerous

If you are a shallow breather, the assistance offered your heart by breathing is reduced, and a slow-down in circulation causes weakness, fatigue, and brain fog from an oxygen deficiency. When you hold your breath, the effect of breathing upon circulation is, of course, lost.

You should never take a deep breath and hold it during heavy exertion. This would completely obstruct the circulation of blood. Here's why: If the muscles of the thorax and the abdomen are contracted while the lungs are filled with air and the glottis (throat) is closed, compression of the lungs and the abdominal organs creates a positive pressure in the thoracic and abdominal cavities. This interferes with the return of venous blood to the heart by compressing the great vein (vena cava) that travels up through the abdomen and the chest. If this compression continues for longer than a few seconds, obstruction of the circulation can cause a *blackout* by reducing the amount of arterial blood being pumped to the brain. If the heart doesn't receive venous blood, it can't pump out arterial blood, and your body won't get enough oxygen.

I have seen many athletes "pass out" while holding their breath during a prolonged exertion. A construction worker who took a deep breath and held it while lifting a heavy beam was seriously injured when he blacked out and fell from a building. Always remember to *exhale* when you make a heavy effort.

THE GOOD AND BAD IN ABDOMINAL BREATHING

Although chest or thoracic breathing is best for aiding the circulation of blood and supplying additional oxygen, it might be a good idea to occasionally breathe deeply into your abdomen. This will assure expansion of the lower lobes of your lungs as well as exercise your diaphragm.

The diaphragm is a sheet of muscle that separates the abdominal organs from the lungs. Each time you inhale, your diaphragm moves downward to increase the size of your chest cavity and to suck air into your lungs. When you are relaxed and rested, it is the diaphragm that does most of the work during breathing—and it functions automatically. When you make a deliberate effort to use only your diaphragm in deep abdominal breathing, pressure against the abdominal organs may interfere with the circulation of blood.

So while you should occasionally practice abdominal breathing, you should not attempt to breathe this way all the time, as recommended by some "breathing experts."

INCREASE YOUR LUNG CAPACITY BY
STRETCHING YOUR CHEST

The greater your chest capacity, the more air you can inhale for a fresh supply of oxygen and the greater the effect of breathing upon circulation. Also, the more lung tissue you have, the more oxygen your blood can absorb with each breath. For this reason, it might be a good idea to take at least one exercise that will stretch your rib cage and strengthen the muscles that lift your ribs.

In addition to expanding your lungs, a regular chest exercise will give you a youthful, prosperous look by improving your posture and increasing your chest size.

When I recommended a special chest-expanding exercise for a 48-year-old salesman who was despondent because of his failure to meet his sales quota, not only did he begin to look better and feel better, but also his sales began to pick up. The change in his physical appearance made him appear more youthful and confident, adding a positive note to his sales presentation.

A barber who practiced the same exercise reported that he had less fatigue and that his legs did not ache nearly as much at the end of the day. "I feel better all over," he said. "I have more energy than I've had in years. That exercise seems to clear my brain so that I can work a little faster. And the more hair I cut the more money I make."

Both of these men literally cashed in on their new-found youthful health and vigor. Good health is essential for success in almost any endeavor. How you feel can have a lot to do with how you get along in this world.

The Isometric Chest Expander

This is an exercise that you can do almost anywhere. And the only movement that takes place is in your chest.

Sit in front of a table and extend your arms straight out in front with your hands palms down on the top of the table. Press down lightly with your hands while inhaling deeply. Lift your chest as high as you can. Make sure that your abdominal muscles stay relaxed.

The downward pressure exerted by your arms will anchor your shoulder girdle so that certain chest muscles can lift your ribs. Try this exercise and see if you aren't able to expand your chest more than usual.

BEWARE OF HYPERVENTILATION

Although you should breathe deeply several times each day, you should not take more than two or three deep breaths at one time unless you are breathless from exertion. Hyperventilation, or forced deep breathing when you don't need additional oxygen, can cause dizziness, nausea, and other symptoms by siphoning too much carbon dioxide out of your blood and constricting the blood vessels around your brain.

In my files, I have the case history of one nervous patient who complained of numbness, irregular heart beat, and dizziness that were caused solely by overbreathing. She was constantly sighing, and when she felt her heart do a "flip flop," she felt that if she didn't breathe deeply she would surely die. When she began to feel a numbness creeping over her body from hyperventilation, she would panic and begin to gasp for air. As a result, she would become so dizzy that she could not even stand without fainting. Her attacks lasted for hours, causing great concern for her family. Her family physician prescribed tranquilizers to calm her down and make her sleep. A careful medical examination had ruled out any obvious organic disease.

When I explained the effects of hyperventilation to this woman, she was able to avoid overbreathing caused by panic. She learned to terminate excessive sighing and anxiety by breathing into a small paper bag for a couple of minutes to restore the balance of carbon dioxide and oxygen in her blood.

Carbon dioxide is a waste product of the body, but a certain amount must be present in the blood to help regulate heart rate and respiration and to dilate blood vessels. Normally, forced deep breathing does not take place unless exercise or exertion has created a need for oxygen and an excessive amount of carbon dioxide has accumulated in the blood. For this reason, a person who wants to practice a prolonged breathing exercise should do so only after building up an oxygen debt by taking a little exercise.

If you jog or swim to strengthen your heart, as suggested in Chapter 9, do your breathing exercises immediately following each workout. Whether you exercise or not, try to breathe deeply at least once every hour of every day. This should be enough to aerate your lungs, stimulate your circulation, and cleanse your blood. Every time you climb a flight of stairs or walk a block or two, expand your chest with as many deep breaths as necessary to satisfy your body's need for oxygen.

HOW TO BREATHE STALE AIR OUT OF YOUR LUNGS

So far, all of the breathing exercises you've learned about

develop only those muscles used during inhalation. It's also important occasionally to practice forced *exhalation.* Actually, it's impossible to empty the lungs completely, since some air remains in the lungs even after a maximum expiration. But each time you exhale and then inhale, the residual stale air is diluted with fresh air. So when you want to clean out your lungs and increase the amount of oxygen in your blood, exhalation can be just as important as inhalation.

When you exhale forcefully, many of the muscles around your chest, back, and abdomen are activated. You can strengthen all of these muscles simply by breathing out until your abdominal muscles are flat and tightly contracted. Your diaphragm will automatically move up into your chest and press most of the air out of your lungs.

If you want to exercise your abdominal muscles by contracting them repeatedly, don't precede each contraction with a deep breath. Just inhale a small amount of air (without lifting your chest) before each contraction. Then exhale as vigorously as you can while tightening your abdominal muscles. Several contractions each day will firm and tone your abdomen as well as force stale air out of your lungs.

SHAVASAN TO RELAX YOUR BODY AND CLEAN YOUR BLOOD

There is some evidence to indicate that shavasan, a Yogi technique of lying on your back and breathing in and out *slowly* for half an hour or so, will relieve headaches, nervousness, and high blood pressure caused by tension. It undoubtedly does so by relaxing muscles and aiding the circulation of blood.

A real estate broker and his wife who tried shavasan reported that they were completely "tranquilized." The husband said that his blood pressure dropped from an abnormally high level to "just above normal." The wife claimed relief from "headaches and anxiety."

If you have enough free time each day to practice shavasan, then do so. It should fit well into your youth-building program. Otherwise, just be sure to get a good night's sleep, which is just one long shavasan.

A WARNING ABOUT SMOKING

Cigarette smoke is greatly damaging to the lungs. It can also suffocate your body. Experiments conducted at the University of California, for example, revealed that ten inhalations of cigarette smoke would close 50 percent of the lung's air passages for about one hour by constricting tiny bronchioles.

Bathing the lungs with smoke can also prevent the exchange of carbon dioxide for oxygen by coating the air sacs with tar. Lung tissue may harden so that it cannot even absorb oxygen. In Chapter 8, you'll learn how the carbon monoxide in cigarette smoke can actually prevent your red blood cells from absorbing oxygen.

If you want to be truly youthful and vigorous, you should not smoke. If you already smoke, then make up your mind to quit *now*. When your lungs and your blood cells have been relieved of the burden of cigarette smoke, a free exchange of carbon dioxide for oxygen will make you feel 100 percent better. Best of all, you'll be less likely to suffer from such crippling diseases as lung cancer, coronary disease, bronchitis, asthma, emphysema, stomach ulcers, and arteriosclerosis. You'll have a better chance of growing old without becoming sick or prematurely senile.

SUMMARY

1. Lifting your chest during a deep breath will aid the circulation of blood as well as expand your lungs.

2. To avoid excessive hyperventilation, don't take more than two or three deep breaths at one time unless you're breathless from exertion.

3. Every time you take a little exercise, practice deep breathing until your body's need for oxygen is satisfied.

4. Don't ever take a deep breath and hold it during a heavy exertion. Always exhale when you contract your abdominal muscles.

5. Practice abdominal breathing occasionally by bulging out your abdomen with a deep inspiration.

6. Try the isometric chest-expanding exercise described in this chapter if you want a bigger chest with a greater lung capacity.

7. Occasionally empty your lungs with a forced expiration by flattening and contracting your abdominal muscles.

8. Lying down and breathing *slowly* for about half an hour will relieve nervous tension and relax muscles as well as aid the circulation of blood.

9. Cigarette smoke interferes with absorption of oxygen by loading the red blood cells with carbon monoxide, by coating the lungs with tar, and by hardening the air sacs.

10. Remember that without iron your blood cannot absorb oxygen, so be sure to read Chapter 8.

8

How to Build Rich, Red Blood for Youthful Health

If you eat properly and observe all the rules of nutrition outlined in Chapter 4, you'll supply your body with all the nutrients it needs to build "healthy" blood. There is reason to believe, however, that the average person could use some additional iron in building solid, bright-red blood cells. *The more iron your blood contains the more oxygen it can transport to youthful, vibrant tissue cells.* Iron also aids in the removal of waste products that must be excreted through the lungs.

Unfortunately, the average person has far less iron in his blood than he needs for superior health. In fact, iron-deficiency anemia is so common that it is considered "normal" for the red blood cells to contain only 80 percent of the amount of iron they're capable of holding. If you want to be truly youthful and vigorous, you should take steps to make sure that the iron content of your blood measures out 100 percent.

Iron-deficiency anemia can cause many symptoms that can mimic a great variety of illnesses. A middle-aged housewife, for example, complaining of headache, fatigue, numbness, and shortness of breath had been told by her family physician that the change of life was making her nervous. Her blood was tested for iron and the reading came out *less* than 70 percent. When she added a few iron-rich foods to her diet, her symptoms vanished. "If I had only known what was wrong five years ago," she said, "I could have saved all those wasted years."

There are undoubtedly many people who could restore their vim and vigor by loading their blood cells with iron. This chapter will tell you everything you need to know to get all the iron *you* need.

BUILDING BETTER HEMOGLOBIN

Most of the iron in your blood combines with a substance called hemoglobin, which is found only in red blood cells. Basically, hemoglobin is composed of protein and iron, but there are many vitamins and minerals that play a part in its formation. The acid in your stomach, for example, dissolves the iron in your foods so that it can be absorbed by your body. But without certain B vitamins, your stomach cannot secrete this acid. Copper must be absorbed along with the iron before it can be used by the body. Folic acid, a B vitamin that is essential for the production of blood cells, cannot be utilized without Vitamin C.

A deficiency in Vitamin B_6 can actually cause anemia. And if an attempt is made to correct this type of anemia by giving more and more iron, serious illness could result.

Even Vitamin E is necessary for the absorption of iron. When there is a deficiency in this vitamin, the red blood cells can be oxidized or destroyed by the oxygen they're supposed to transport.

In addition to forming the framework of blood cells, protein forms "plasma protein," which stores amino acids and forms antibodies to combat disease. Even fibrinogen, the sticky stuff that forms clots to stop bleeding, is made of protein.

So no matter what you hear about the importance of iron in your diet, remember that a *balanced diet* comes first.

Actually, your blood is about 80 percent water, 18 percent protein, and only two percent chemicals. But every last milligram of all the vitamins and minerals in your blood, especially the iron, is essential to long life and a youthful appearance.

THE IMPORTANCE OF IRON IN COMBATING
THE AGING PROCESS

When the blood is deficient in iron, the skin, nails, and membranes become ghostly pale. In extreme cases, the eyeballs may be bluish in color. In pronounced cases of iron-deficiency anemia, an oxygen deficiency in the blood can cause such symptoms as fatigue, faintness, headache, dizziness, shortness of breath, stomach and intestinal trouble, ringing in the ears, spots before the eyes, and so on. Interest in sex may also be diminished.

Uncorrected anemia can even cause premature aging by wrinkling the skin and turning the hair gray. Nails may become brittle, flat or even spoon-shaped. Resistance against infection and disease may be so low that the individual is constantly suffering from a "secondary illness."

Your body also needs iron to construct its tissues, but most of the symptoms associated with anemia are caused by an *oxygen deficiency.* The iron-deficient blood cells simply cannot carry enough oxygen to meet the needs of the body.

Obviously, you cannot afford to be deficient in iron if you want to live a long, youthful life. If you think that you might be anemic, ask your doctor for a test that will measure the amount of iron in your blood. If he says that your hemoglobin is less than 80 percent, you may need an iron supplement.

Increase your intake of natural iron-rich foods whether you think you are anemic or not. Try to build up your hemoglobin so that it measures 100 percent in its iron content. If you can do this by eating the foods provided by nature, you'll benefit in many ways, and you'll look better and feel better.

A 35-year-old secretary who was "tired" all the time restored her energy and changed her complexion from a sickly pale to youthful pink by eating liver and wheat germ. She gave up her cola and sandwich diet for a balanced diet of wholesome, natural foods. All of her symptoms of anemia disappeared, and her mood changed from one of depression and irritability to one of sparkling vivaciousness. "I didn't know eating could be so important," she said. "I just thought I was getting old."

In another case, a "skinny" dental assistant who had fainted a couple of times while helping the dentist blamed it on the sight of blood until she found out she was anemic. When her diet was corrected, her faintness disappeared and her appetite improved. She began to gain weight and soon had a very shapely figure.

So you can see that anemia, like any other abnormal state of health, can have far-reaching effects on both your mind and your body. To be youthful for a long life, you have to make sure that you have good all-around health.

BUILDING NEW BLOOD CELLS

There are normally about 35 trillion red blood cells in the human body. The life of a healthy cell is normally about three or four months. This means that your bone marrow and your liver must constantly be producing new blood cells in order to maintain a healthy volume of blood. Your bone marrow alone builds about one billion red blood cells every minute. Your liver does a good job of breaking down old, wornout cells and salvaging their iron. But without a rich supply of iron from natural foods, the blood cells would become so thin and anemic that they would absorb very little oxygen when they pass through your lungs. They would also break easily when they are pumped through your heart.

There are normally about four grams of iron in the blood. If you are a robust and healthy person, however, you may have more red blood cells than the average person, and your hemoglobin may contain more iron. Furthermore, your blood cells are probably thick and strong enough to withstand considerable stress and to carry a maximum amount of oxygen.

FOOD SOURCES OF IRON

Most natural foods contain some iron, but excessive use of refined foods has deprived many people of the amount of iron they need for a long and energetic life. Loss of Vitamins B and E in the processing of foods has also contributed to the development of iron-deficiency anemia. Try to eat a variety of fresh, wholesome foods whenever possible. It's not enough just to take an iron pill. Remember that practically everything you eat contributes to the absorption and use of iron in building red blood cells.

Whole wheat flour, lima beans, kidney beans, soybeans, peanuts, dark molasses, fresh fruits, green leafy vegetables, egg yolk, muscle meats, kidneys, and dried peaches and apricots are good sources of iron.

Liver is probably the best source of iron, and it's the best "medicine" you can get for correcting iron-deficiency anemia. Gizzards are also rich in iron. Try to eat liver at least once a week. Properly prepared, it's delicious as well as nutritious.

Contrary to popular opinion, raisins are not the richest source of iron. Actually, they contain less iron than egg yolk, spinach, peas, beans, and other foods that are only moderately rich in iron. Raisins are a fine, nutritious food, but don't try to rely upon them for your daily iron requirement.

How Much Iron Do You Need?

According to most nutritionists, you need about 15 milligrams of iron each day for good health. For youthful health and vigor, however, you probably need more iron than that amount.

A two-ounce piece of pork liver contains about 15 mg. of iron; one-half cup of wheat germ, about 6.4 mg.; one tablespoonful of brewer's yeast, about 2 mg.; five dried apricots, 4.6 mg.; and one-half cup of parsley, 9.6 mg. So you can see that it shouldn't be too difficult to get more than enough iron from the foods you eat.

If you would like to supplement your diet with a little extra iron (in addition to that you get from liver and green leafy vegetables), sprinkle your foods with wheat germ or brewer's yeast. Both are rich in iron as well as vitamins and minerals.

Parsley is so rich in iron that you should try to use it in all of your salads—along with bean sprouts when they are available.

Don't forget that protein is just as essential as iron in building blood. Always try to include meat, fish, or poultry in your daily diet. Liver is rich in both protein and iron, and it's low in saturated fat. If you're concerned about the fat in your diet, turn to Chapter 9 for a list of high-protein, low-fat foods.

SMOKING AND SYMPTOMS OF ANEMIA

Many heavy smokers suffer from symptoms of anemia—not necessarily because they are deficient in iron, but because the effects of cigarette smoke interfere with the body's absorption of oxygen.

Filling the lungs with smoke crowds out fresh, clean air, so that the red blood cells absorb carbon monoxide instead of oxygen. For some reason, hemoglobin has a greater affinity for carbon monoxide than for oxygen. And once carbon monoxide has locked onto a blood cell, it is reluctant to let it go. It may, in fact, take several days for red blood cells to get rid of the carbon monoxide they pick up from the smoke of a single cigarette. This means that if you smoke "occasionally," you cannot expect to cleanse your blood by breathing deeply between cigarettes.

It takes only about 21 seconds for the circulation of blood to complete a circuit through the body. Most of the red blood cells in the body can be exposed to carbon monoxide in the lungs in less time than it takes to smoke only one cigarette—and the symptoms that result may persist for days.

A mechanic who worked in a poorly ventilated garage complained of weakness, nausea, headache, dizziness, and other symptoms that persisted over weekends and holidays. When blood tests revealed a normal iron content, he was subjected to a variety of expensive medical tests. When no organic disease could be found, he was told that his trouble might be emotional and that perhaps he was unhappy with his job. A week or two after he changed jobs, his symptoms vanished—not because of a change in his state of mind but because he was finally breathing clean, fresh air. All of the carbon monoxide in his blood was eventually replaced by oxygen.

A chain smoker who keeps his lungs filled with smoke and his blood cells loaded with carbon monoxide may suffer from carbon dioxide poisoning as well as from oxygen deficiency. This can cause depression, drowsiness, and mental confusion. It may also cause premature aging. Hemoglobin normally unloads oxygen in the tissues and picks up carbon dioxide for elimination through the lungs, but it can't fulfill either of these functions when it is loaded with carbon monoxide.

EXERCISE INCREASES THE NUMBER OF RED BLOOD CELLS

Persons who take a little regular exercise may have more

red blood cells than a sedentary person. The reason for this, of course, is that an increased need for oxygen in the muscles stimulates the production of the blood cells needed to transport the oxygen.

Living and working at a high altitude also increases the number of red blood cells. The low partial pressure of the oxygen in the air forces the body to produce more blood cells to absorb more oxygen. There are some athletes who believe that training at a high altitude will temporarily improve their performance at a lower altitude by increasing the oxygen-carrying capacity of their blood.

Why not spend your next vacation in the mountains? It might give you a temporary boost when you return to work.

PERNICIOUS ANEMIA CAN BE DEADLY

Most forms of iron-deficiency anemia can be corrected by making simple changes in the diet. In pernicious anemia, however, which is characterized by undeveloped red blood cells, there are deficiencies in the body that cannot be corrected by diet alone. There may be adequate iron in the diet, but it cannot be absorbed because of an absence of hydrochloric acid in the stomach. A substance needed for the absorption of Vitamin B_{12} is also missing. As a result, the bone marrow is unable to manufacture an adequate number of red blood cells. The missing vitamin also deprives the nervous system of adequate nourishment.

Doctors have discovered that folic acid, one of the B vitamins, will relieve fatigue and other symptoms of anemia by increasing the production of red blood cells. But if the Vitamin B_{12} deficiency is allowed to continue, the victim may be crippled by damaged nerves. For this reason, folic acid is now sold only by prescription just to make sure that pernicious anemia doesn't go undetected in routine blood examinations.

When pernicious anemia is discovered, it must be treated

by a physician who can give injections of Vitamin B_{12}. Hydrochloric acid may also be given so that the stomach can absorb iron. In some cases, for example, one or two teaspoons of diluted hydrochloric acid may be mixed in one-half glass of water so that it can be sipped through a glass straw with each meal.

A WARNING FOR VEGETARIANS

Vitamin B_{12} is found almost exclusively in animal protein. A vegetarian who does not include milk, cheese, fish, or eggs in his diet might acquire pernicious anemia from a dietary deficiency of this important vitamin.

Yeast, wheat germ, and soybeans contain traces of B_{12}, but not enough to meet the needs of the body. Most vegetables do contain folic acid, however, and this is one reason why a pure vegetarian diet might be dangerous. The folic acid might mask symptoms of pernicious anemia until the B_{12} deficiency does some permanent damage to the nervous system. If you don't want to eat meat, you should eat fish or poultry—or at least include milk, eggs, and cheese.

Fatigue, weakness, tingling hands and feet, and a sore, smooth, beefy-red tongue may be early signs of pernicious anemia or a Vitamin B_{12} deficiency. If you experience any of these symptoms, ask your doctor to count your red cells and measure their iron content.

OTHER CAUSES OF ANEMIA

There are so many causes and types of anemia that only a physician can distinguish one from another in selecting proper treatment. Blood loss, infection, exposure to pesticides, disease, drugs, and inherited factors, for example, must sometimes be considered. Food additives and synthetic foods may indirectly cause anemia by leading to a vitamin shortage. Excessive use of alkalies can neutralize the acid secreted by the stomach to prevent absorption of iron.

Some forms of anemia are caused by a shortage of blood cells rather than by a shortage of iron. In these cases, there may be disease in the blood-making organs.

It is your responsibility to prevent anemia of a *dietary* origin. You can do this easily by eating fresh, wholesome foods that are rich in iron, and B vitamins, along with a balanced diet that contains all the essential food elements. You can benefit from the suggestions offered in this chapter whether you think you are anemic or not. It is, in fact, essential that you follow them if you want to be exceptionally youthful and vigorous.

If you develop any of the symptoms of anemia in spite of good eating habits, you should have a good medical checkup.

SUMMARY

1. A good, balanced diet contributes protein, vitamins, and minerals that are essential in the formation of blood.

2. Increase your intake of such iron-rich foods as liver, brewer's yeast, whole wheat products, and green leafy vegetables so that your blood will be rich and red.

3. Most of the iron in your blood combines with protein to form hemoglobin, which transports oxygen from your lungs to your tissues. An iron deficiency results in an oxygen deficiency, which can cause fatigue, shortness of breath, and other symptoms that contribute to premature aging.

4. Carbon monoxide from cigarette smoke can combine with hemoglobin to prevent absorption of oxygen.

5. Regular exercise increases the number of red blood cells in order to meet the body's demand for additional oxygen.

6. Since stomach acid is necessary for the absorption of iron, excessive use of alkalies can result in iron-deficiency anemia.

7. Pernicious anemia can be caused by a "bad stomach" that does not produce enough hydrochloric acid and does not absorb iron and Vitamin B_{12}.

8. A vegetarian who does not include milk, eggs, cheese, or fish in his diet could develop pernicious anemia from a Vitamin B_{12} deficiency.

9. Remember that there are many causes of anemia, such as blood loss, infection, drug use, and so on, that cannot be corrected by diet alone.

10. Fatigue, flat nails, tingling hands and feet, a sore mouth and tongue, and unusual paleness of skin and mucous membranes may be early signs of a serious form of anemia.

9

How to Make Your Heart Last 100 Youthful Years or Longer

Randy C. was a struggling business man. At the age of 42, he had just leased a restaurant that showed every indication of being a big success. But attention to the business would require long hours and hard work. With two children in high school and one in college, he could not afford another failure. So Randy worked hard, and his enthusiasm increased as his business grew better.

"Now maybe I'll be able to buy a few things for my family," he said hopefully. "I've never even been able to take them on a decent vacation."

The next day, Randy fell dead in his restaurant. He had died of a heart attack—in the prime of his life.

HEART DISEASE: THE MOST COMMON CAUSE OF DEATH

About half of all deaths in the United States are caused by heart disease. Coronary occlusion, or a clot in one of the arteries supplying the heart muscle, is the most common cause of death in men in their middle forties. Of all the diseases the human body is subject to, none is more likely to kill before middle age than heart disease—and usually without warning.

The heart is a tough and durable organ. When it is strong and healthy, it can easily outlast the other organs of the body. Why, then, are so many people dying of heart disease today? Why are the average person's arteries clogged with fat before he reaches middle age?

Prior to about 1900, death from clogging of the coronary arteries was rare. In fact, one leading heart specialist says that coronary thrombosis was unheard of when he graduated from medical school in 1911. Medical literature indicates that death from coronary occlusion became more and more common after 1912.

An increased amount of fat and cholesterol in the blood is the apparent cause of most fatal heart attacks. But there are several theories as to where this fat comes from.

In observing the changes in eating habits since 1900, it seems likely that an increased consumption of refined and artificial foods has contributed something to the development of heart disease as we know it today. The use of sugar and white-flour products has increased tremendously over the past half century. Both of these fat-building foods increase the amount of cholesterol in the blood. Furthermore, the refining of such foods has eliminated certain vitamins, minerals, and other elements that are known to be essential to good heart health.

It is the consensus of most medical men at the present time, however, that animal fat is the biggest source of excess blood fat. For this reason, most diets for heart patients restrict the use of fat meats and dairy products.

FAT ARTERIES CAN AGE YOUR BODY

The accumulation of fat and cholesterol inside the arteries is called *atherosclerosis*. In addition to forming a thrombus or clot that can break loose and lodge in a coronary (heart) artery to cause a coronary occlusion, a build-up of fatty sludge in the blood can deprive the heart and other tissues of adequate blood and oxygen. It can also raise blood pressure and cause premature aging.

Arteriosclerosis, in which the walls of the arteries are hardened by fat, commonly causes mental confusion in elderly persons by depriving the brain of adequate oxygen.

The amount of fat and cholesterol in the blood can be reduced by making a few simple dietary changes. There are, however, other measures that must be taken if you want to keep your heart muscle strong and your coronary arteries youthful and healthy. Exercise and emotional tranquility, for example, are also important, as you'll learn later in this chapter.

HOW YOU CAN REDUCE THE AMOUNT OF HARMFUL FAT IN YOUR DIET

Although any kind of hard fat in the blood can clog the arteries, cholesterol seems to be the biggest offender in coronary occlusion. For this reason, an attempt is usually made to eliminate all dietary cholesterol.

Actually, cholesterol is an important ingredient of just about every tissue and organ in the body, including the brain. It can be synthesized in the liver and in the tissues, but a certain amount must be supplied in the foods we eat. High-cholesterol foods, however, should be drastically reduced in the diets of inactive persons who are 40 years of age or older. *Sugar and refined foods should be completely eliminated.*

If you can learn to balance animal fat and vegetable oils in your diet, you can prevent hard fat from accumulating in your arteries. You can actually dissolve cholesterol deposits that might be interfering with the flow of blood through your body.

Balancing Animal Fat and Vegetable Fat

Basically, there are two types of fat in the food you eat—saturated and unsaturated.

Saturated fat is a "hard fat" that tends to harden inside your arteries, just as it does in a can.

Unsaturated fat is a "soft fat" that remains liquid at all times, even at a low temperature.

Most of the saturated fat we put into our mouths comes from foods of animal origin. The fat on meat, for example, is made up almost entirely of saturated fat, and it's so hard that it remains solid even at a high temperature. Eggs, whole milk, yellow cheese, butter, and lard are also rich in saturated fat and cholesterol. Fish and chicken, however, are fairly low in saturated fat.

Vegetables, grains, seeds, and nuts contain unsaturated fat. Cold-pressed vegetable oils are especially rich in unsaturated or soft fat, and they contain fatty acids that are essential to good health. Linoleic, linolenic, and arachidonic acids, for example, cannot be manufactured by the body, and must be supplied by vegetable oil. Without the essential fatty acids, the fat in your blood would quickly solidify.

In order to make sure that you don't have too much hard fat in your blood, you should trim all fat from the meat you eat and increase your intake of fruits and vegetables. Try to eat more chicken and fish, and less beef and pork. Bake or broil your meats. If you boil meat in soup, chill the soup in the refrigerator and then skim off the hard surface fat before serving. Drink skim milk instead of whole milk. Eat cottage cheese instead of yellow cheese. "Processed" cheeses should be eliminated altogether.

Use vegetable oils in your cooking and on your salads. Oil from corn, peanuts, wheat, soybeans, or the safflower, for example, is rich in the essential fatty acids or soft fat. Don't fry your foods, however, even if you use vegetable oil, since high heat might destroy some of the essential fatty acids.

The more hard fat you eat, the more vegetable oil you need to emulsify the fat in your blood. But if you don't cut down on the total amount of fat in your diet, beginning with meat fat, sugar, and white-flour products, you'll be greatly overweight—and this by itself can place a strain on your heart and age you. Actually, the amount of fat in your diet should be reduced to less than 30 percent of your total food intake, with about two-thirds of the fat coming from vegetable sources.

A 38-year-old overweight school teacher who discovered during a routine physical examination that he had a high blood cholesterol count was placed on the type of low-fat diet recommended in this chapter. By the time his blood cholesterol fell back to normal, he had lost considerable weight, and the fatigue and swollen ankles caused by a "weak heart" completely disappeared. So for your heart's sake, as well as for your body's sake, you should eliminate all dietary sources of hard fat; that is, of course, if you want to be youthfully fit and live a long life.

Hard Vegetable Fat Is Harmful Fat

Vegetable oils that have been hydrogenated, or hardened by a chemical process that links hydrogen with the fatty acids, contain harmful saturated fat. Margarine, for example, is made from hardened vegetable oil, and should be eliminated along with animal fat.

Many processed or refined foods contain hardened vegetable oil. The oil in most commercial peanut butter, for example, has been hydrogenated to retard spoilage and to give it a longer life on the shelf of a grocery store. Read the labels on the cans and packages you buy. Avoid those that contain hard fat. Try to steer clear of processed foods.

LECITHIN WILL DISSOLVE THE CHOLESTEROL IN YOUR BLOOD

Most natural foods that contain cholesterol also contain

lecithin, a fat-like substance that will emulsify the cholesterol so that it can be utilized by the body. Lecithin is also manufactured in the liver along with cholesterol, and, like cholesterol, is essential to the function of every cell in the body. When the body is healthy and the diet is properly balanced, there will be a balance between cholesterol and lecithin.

Unfortunately, many of the refined foods we eat today are rich in saturated fat and deficient in lecithin. Processing destroys lecithin and the essential fatty acids. This contributes to atherosclerosis by leaving the cholesterol free to clump together and accumulate inside the arteries.

When adequate lecithin is added to the diet, the lumpy cholesterol in the blood stream breaks up into tiny particles so that it can circulate and be absorbed.

Lecithin can be obtained from egg yolk, seeds, nuts, grains, and liver, as well as from some vegetables. Soybeans and avocados, for example, are rich sources of lecithin. The body can manufacture lecithin from vegetable oil that contains the essential fatty acids. Most drug stores sell pure soybean lecithin that may be purchased in powder, tablets, or granules without a prescription. All you have to do is ask for it.

Experiments indicate that atherosclerosis will not occur if there is adequate lecithin in the diet. So if you cannot stick to a diet of natural foods that are low in saturated fat, you should supplement your diet with lecithin.

A 40-year-old theater manager who refused to quit eating bacon and butter had a recurrence of chest pain everytime he quit taking lecithin. A chiropractor friend of mine who had "heart trouble" also complained of chest pain when he didn't take his lecithin. In both of these cases a rapid accumulation of cholesterol in the arteries simply restricted the circulation of blood to the heart muscle. When they took their lecithin, however, the cholesterol was dissolved so that it could circulate freely through the arteries.

Remember that most natural foods that have not been overly heated or processed contain some lecithin. This is why you should eat your foods raw whenever possible, especially seeds, nuts, fruits, vegetables, and grains. When you do cook meats and vegetables, use as little heat as possible for as short a time as possible.

Some people have a high blood cholesterol count that does not seem to be related to a bad diet. In these cases, a lecithin supplement may be needed to balance abnormal body chemistry. As you'll learn later in this chapter, however, cigarettes, coffee, alcohol, lack of exercise, and emotional strain can increase the amount of cholesterol in the blood.

Your Body Needs B Vitamins to Produce Lecithin

It's well known that the B vitamins choline, inositol, and pyridoxine help to prevent hard fat from accumulating in the arteries. Without these important vitamins, the liver cannot produce lecithin. Choline can be made from "left over" protein in the liver, but it is essential that the diet contain foods that are rich in *all* of the B vitamins.

Liver, wheat germ, and brewer's yeast can supply both protein and B vitamins, and they're low in saturated fat. If you can eat some of all three of these "wonder foods" during the week, your body should get all the B vitamins it needs, along with a generous supply of lecithin.

Brewer's yeast and wheat germ are so valuable in building all-around good health that it might be a good idea to use them as daily supplements.

Wheat germ can be eaten as cereal or sprinkled over foods. Try to add it to bread, biscuits, meat loaf, and other foods that are cooked at home. Most grocery stores sell toasted wheat germ. You can get raw wheat germ in health food stores.

Brewer's yeast may be taken in tablet form, or it may be purchased as a powder for stirring in fruit juice or sprinkling over foods. Check with your local health food store or drug store. Be sure to get *brewer's yeast* and not raw baker's yeast. The latter contains live yeast plants that will steal B vitamins rather than supply them.

The Controversy About Eggs

Egg yolk contains a considerable amount of cholesterol. It also contains lecithin. Some doctors advise their patients not to eat eggs. Others say that the lecithin in the egg counteracts the cholesterol.

It does not seem likely that a food as wholesome and complete as an egg should be eliminated from the diet of the average person. The body needs some cholesterol in addition to what it can manufacture. When there is not enough cholesterol in the diet, the liver might overcompensate and produce more than the body can use. Besides, the egg contains many valuable nutrients, including Vitamin A, which has been removed from skim milk, cottage cheese, and other "low fat" products made from skim milk. It's also rich in methionine, an amino acid that the body can convert into choline (the B vitamin that lowers blood fat and contributes to the formation of lecithin).

You should probably eat at least one egg each day—more if you like them and you are cutting down on other sources of hard fat in your diet. You may, of course, eat all the egg white you want. A fertile egg (one that can be hatched) may be more nutritious than a non-fertile egg. So try to get your eggs from hens that enjoy the company of a rooster.

Be careful not to overcook your eggs. Too much heat might destroy the lecithin in the yolk. Try to leave the yolk slightly runny if you can eat it that way. Soft-boiled eggs cooked in their shell are best. If you fry your eggs, use vegetable oil and low heat.

It is not generally advisable to eat raw eggs. Uncooked egg white contains a toxic substance called "avidin," which prevents the body from absorbing the B vitamin biotin.

VITAMIN E PROTECTS THE ESSENTIAL FATTY ACIDS

When the diet is deficient in Vitamin E, the oxygen in the blood can destroy the essential fatty acids, and the need for oxygen increases in all the tissues of the body, including the heart muscle. In addition to placing additional work on the heart by forcing it to pump more blood, the loss of the essential fatty acids allows fat and cholesterol to harden inside the arteries.

Vegetable oil helps dissolve hard fat, but the more oil you take, the more Vitamin E you need to supply protection for the essential fatty acids. Most vegetable oils contain Vitamin E, but there may not be enough E to go around if the diet is rich in hard fat and the arteries are already diseased.

How to Get Additional Vitamin E for a Strong Young Heart

Wheat germ oil is the richest source of Vitamin E, but it should not completely replace seeds, nuts, whole grain products, green leafy vegetables, and other natural foods that contain this vitamin. If you're on a low-fat diet that includes generous use of fruits and vegetables, two tablespoons of wheat germ oil each day (two teaspoons at each meal) should supply adequate Vitamin E along with unsaturated fat.

Two or three nights each week, I eat a big bowl of shredded wheat mixed with wheat germ, raisins, diced apple, a sliced banana, skim milk, and honey. This makes a delicious high-protein, low-fat meal that literally melts the fat in my arteries. I usually top it off with raw nuts or seeds and an orange.

All vegetable oils, except coconut oil and olive oil, contain unsaturated fat along with Vitamin E. If you supplement your diet with wheat germ oil, however, you won't have to use any other vegetable oil except for cooking purposes.

Persons who have heart trouble may have to supplement their diet with Vitamin E capsules in order to avoid taking an excessive amount of vegetable oil. Too much Vitamin E supplied by a high-powered supplement, however, might be harmful to a rheumatic heart. Check with your doctor. Turn back to Chapter 4 for additional information on Vitamin E.

A BLOOD TEST FOR CHOLESTEROL

If you'd like to find out how much cholesterol you have in your blood, ask your family physician for a cholesterol test. A small amount of blood drawn from your arm will tell the story. If your doctor reports that you have less than 180 milligrams, your cholesterol is not excessive. Most doctors consider any reading between 150 and 250 to be normal. But if you eat properly, you'll have less blood cholesterol than the average person.

Many people who die of heart attacks caused by athero-sclerosis have a cholesterol count that ranges from 250 to 450 milligrams. A high blood fat without an associated high blood cholesterol is also dangerous, and should be corrected by diet and exercise.

AN EYE TEST FOR HEART DISEASE

Many elderly persons who suffer from an accumulation of hard fat in their arteries show some evidence of the disease in their eyes. There may be a white or grayish ring circling the inside border of the iris (the colored portion of the eye), for example, or there may be yellow fatty accumulations in the skin around the eyes. (See Figure 9-1.)

If you're under 45 years of age and you can see such fat in or around your eyes, you may be aging prematurely from a bad diet. And chances are your arteries are already badly clogged with fat and cholesterol.

If you begin now to observe the eating tips outlined in this chapter, you may be able to dissolve the hard fat in your arteries before any damage to your heart takes place.

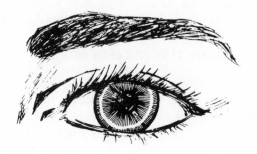

Figure 9-1 *Arcus senilis may be a sign of premature aging.*

THE DANGERS OF CIGARETTES, COFFEE, AND ALCOHOL

The use of cigarettes, coffee, and alcohol is so common today that most people do not realize that they are powerful drugs that can have harmful effects on the body. Excessive use of these products can be just as bad or worse than eating improperly. (See Figure 9-2.)

Cigarettes

Nicotine speeds the heart rate, constricts blood vessels, and destroys Vitamin C in the blood. It can also raise blood cholesterol by stimulating the adrenal glands. And there is now some evidence to indicate that absorption of carbon monoxide by red blood cells contributes to a build-up of fat in the arteries.

A deficiency in Vitamin C caused by heavy smoking might permit a small blood vessel to break and form a clot that could travel to the heart and lodge in a coronary artery. If you combine all of the effects of cigarette smoking with atherosclerosis or heart disease, you have a guaranteed formula for premature death.

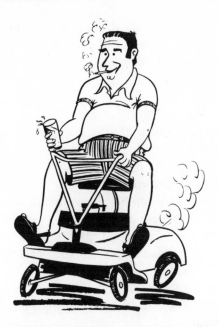

Figure 9-2. *Alcohol, cigarettes, and inadequate exercise contribute greatly to death
caused by heart disease.*

Obviously, the pleasure of puffing on a cigarette isn't
worth the risk, even for a person with healthy arteries and a
strong heart.

Coffee and Cola

The caffeine in coffee and cola drinks can also constrict
blood vessels, increase the heart rate, and stimulate the
adrenal glands. This overworks the heart and starts a chain
reaction that lowers blood sugar and raises blood fat.

I wouldn't deny a coffee lover his morning cup of coffee,
but no one should drink more than two or three cups of
coffee each day.

Coffee is such a powerful stimulant that it can be used as a
drug. One cup of coffee, for example, is sometimes effective

in relieving pain caused by dilated and throbbing arteries in certain types of headaches. Persons who become *addicted* to caffeine, however, may develop a headache when they don't have their usual cup of coffee.

Alcohol

Alcohol is a vasodilator; that is, it *dilates* the arteries rather than constricting them. For this reason, some doctors recommend an occasional drink to improve circulation in certain types of circulatory disorders.

It's important to remember, however, that whenever calories are supplied by alcohol, the calories in food are stored as fat in the tissues. Important B vitamins are destroyed, weakening the nervous system and the heart and interfering with the metabolism of fat.

An occasional social drink may do no harm, but don't be pressured by the cocktail cult into having a drink each day or before each meal.

EMOTIONAL STRAIN CAN KILL YOU

Did you ever notice how hard your heart pounds when you get very nervous? It's a very uncomfortable feeling that cannot be tolerated for very long.

When exercise increases your heart rate, your heart becomes stronger and you feel refreshed and invigorated. But when your heart thumps in response to fear or emotional distress, it leaves you weak and exhausted.

An occasional fright or bout with tension will not damage a healthy heart. When you are subjected to constant tension or emotional harassment, however, your heart may be damaged by harmful nerve impulses that constrict the coronary arteries and reduce the flow of blood to the heart muscle. Stress also increases the amount of fat in the blood, which tends to clog the narrowed arteries.

Nutritionists say that unrelieved emotional stress drains

the body of the nutrients it needs to prevent the formation of clots in the blood. Add cigarettes and a high-fat diet to this and the odds are in favor of a sudden heart attack.

Many high-strung, emotional, and overworked individuals suffer from *angina pectoris,* a heart pain caused by nervous constriction of the coronary arteries. I know one man who experiences chest pain each day in fulfilling his duties as a corporation executive. Just imagine what damage this might do to his heart if he does not find some way to relieve his tension.

You don't have to be a victim of chronic nervous tension. If you can't solve all of your problems, face them and then try to forget them at the end of each day. Participate in sports, recreation, or some other entertaining pastime. Set aside a portion of each day for complete relaxation. Exercise will relieve nervous tension, and it will lower blood fat, dilate blood vessels, and increase the flow of blood to the heart muscle—just the reverse of the effects of nervous tension.

Remember that all work and no play can make Jack a *dead* boy.

A SPECIAL BATH TO RELAX YOUR HEART

If you think your heart is being overworked by nervous tension, you might want to try a special carbon dioxide bath that will slow your heart rate and normalize your blood pressure while aiding the circulation of blood.

Mix five to eight pounds of salt into 40 gallons of warm water. Then add one-half pound of sodium bicarbonate and six to eight large tablets of sodium sulfate. Distribute the tablets over a rubber sheet in the bottom of the tub. (The purpose of the sheet is to prevent corrosive action on the bathtub.)

When the water begins to bubble, lie quietly in the tub and allow the bubbles to accumulate on your skin. Absorption of the carbon dioxide gas will dilate the blood vessels in your skin and give it a bright red glow.

Follow the bath with a rest period of about two hours so that your heart and your arteries can obtain full benefit from their relaxed condition.

"That carbon dioxide bath really helps me," said a 37-year-old bank clerk. "When my blood pressure starts rising and my nerves start getting on edge from handling all those accounts, I find the bath soothing and relaxing."

Try it yourself and see if it won't eliminate the anxiety, the muscle tightness, the headache, or the palpitating heart rate that usually accompanies functional hypertension or nervous tension. These tensions relentlessly make you look older.

EXERCISE WILL STRENGTHEN YOUR HEART

If you want to make sure that your heart will last 100 years or longer, you should take a little regular exercise. A good diet will keep your heart healthy, but you must make a special effort to strengthen your heart muscle.

You can't strain a normal heart, since the skeletal muscles and the lungs will usually "give out" before the heart "gives up." It may be difficult or impossible, however, to be sure that the architecture of your heart and its blood vessels is perfectly normal. The only way that you can be sure of protecting your heart from strain is to strengthen it with regular exercise. Even a defective heart can withstand stress if its walls are thick and strong. A weak and defective heart, however, could be easily strained by prolonged, unaccustomed exertion. Once a "bad heart" has been strained, its walls become thin and flabby from overstretching—and they stay that way.

There's another important reason why you should exercise your heart. If you follow the dietary suggestions outlined in this chapter, your arteries won't be clogged with cholesterol or fat. If you don't exercise, however, your coronary arteries may be too small to supply your heart muscle with adequate blood in an emergency.

When you exercise your heart by forcing it to pump additional blood and oxygen to your skeletal muscles, the blood supply to the heart muscle also increases. This *widens* the coronary arteries and opens tiny capillaries inside the heart muscle. New blood vessels are formed, so that if a clot should clog one artery there will be enough "extra" arteries to keep the heart muscle supplied with adequate blood. Of course, the larger your coronary arteries are the less the chance that one of them will be closed by a clot or a lump of cholesterol.

Doctors who performed an autopsy on the body of an active distance runner who died at the age of 85 found that although his arteries had hardened to some extent, his coronary arteries were more than large enough to keep his heart muscle supplied with plenty of blood. His heart was, in fact, "younger" than the heart of the average 40-year-old man.

Exercise Reduces Blood Fat

In addition to widening coronary arteries, *regular exercise will reduce the amount of fat and cholesterol in your blood.* This is a medically documented fact, not a theory. Some doctors have observed that persons who take plenty of exercise do not develop a high blood cholesterol, no matter what they eat.

Just to be on the safe side, however, you should watch your diet as well as take regular exercise. If you are a big eater and you cannot resist eating certain high-fat foods, it's absolutely imperative that you take some form of exercise. Vegetable oil and lecithin may keep hard fat from accumulating in your arteries, but it won't prevent fat from being stored in your tissues.

Regular exercise will prevent a build-up of body fat, and it will "program" your metabolism for quick disposal of excess calories. A person who exercises, for example, can take in proportionately more calories without gaining weight than a person who doesn't exercise.

Recreational Exercise Is Best

Any exercise that increases heart rate and respiration is a good heart exercise. Endurance-type exercise involving use of the legs is undoubtedly best, since the big muscles of the thighs and hips create a great demand for oxygen-rich blood.

Walking is a fairly good exercise, but it's not nearly as effective as jogging, swimming, riding a bicycle, or jumping a rope. Such a recreational "leg sports" as tennis or basketball are great for exercising the heart. (See Figure 9-3.)

If you prefer *walking,* try to walk at a brisk enough pace to make you a little breathless. If you are not accustomed to walking, however, walk slowly for only a few blocks to begin with. As you become better conditioned, slowly increase the speed and distance of your walking. A short walk each day will do wonders in activating the chemical processes that slow the aging process.

If you'd like to start a *jogging* program, don't do so until you have first spent a few weeks walking. Then alternately walk and jog until you are able to jog a block or two. Don't push yourself. Stop if you experience any pain or discomfort. Each time you jog, you'll be able to jog a little further without any unusual distress. Such a progressive program will give your heart muscle time to develop along with your skeletal muscles. (See Figure 9-4.)

Caution: It's never a good idea for an unconditioned person to test his endurance by seeing how far or how fast he can run. Forget about the 10-minute test that some popular jogging programs use to classify beginners. Always begin your jogging lightly and progressively.

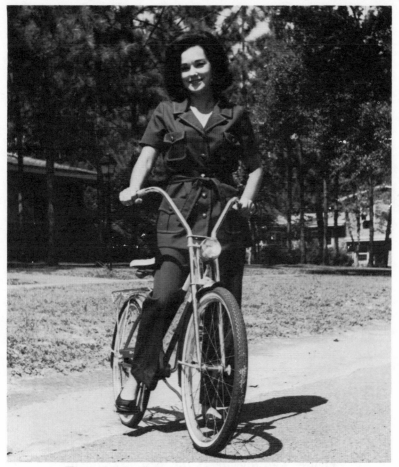

Figure 9-3. *Bicycle riding is a good example of recreational endurance-type exercise.*

Don't ever push yourself to the point of acute distress. Even after you become accustomed to jogging, a mile or two will be adequate if you aren't training for an athletic event.

If you don't have time to exercise every day, try to exercise every other day, or at least twice a week. Once a week or less is not often enough to condition your skeletal muscles, much less your heart muscle. In fact, once-a-week

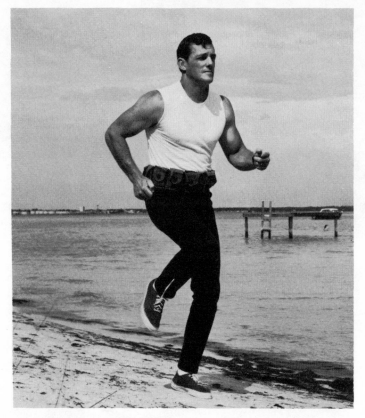

Figure 9-4. *Jogging is the best exercise for the heart muscle.*

exercise may do more harm than good by creating muscle soreness and filling the blood with waste products.

Whatever type of exercise you do, make sure that it's something you enjoy doing. Then try to do it for the rest of your life. If you can keep your heart strong and your muscles toned, you'll feel young and look young, and you'll live longer.

If you're interested in building exceptional heart and

muscle strength for participation in athletics, you can get the information you want from my book *Muscle Training for Athletes,* published by Parker Publishing Company of West Nyack, New York.

CHECK YOUR CONDITION WITH A PULSE-RATE TEST

Step on and off a 12-inch stool for 30 seconds. If your heart rate increases more than 20 to 30 beats per minute and does not return to normal after one minute of rest, you may be physically unfit.

Or try running in place for one minute and then lie down and take your pulse. If your heart rate is not less than 100 beats per minute, your heart is working harder than it should.

Once your heart and your muscles have been conditioned by regular exercise, your pulse rate will be lower and it will return to normal faster following exercise or exertion. There will also be less difference between your pulse rates taken while standing and while lying down. Normally, your heart rate should not increase over 15 beats per minute when you stand after lying on your back for several minutes. When there is a big difference between standing and reclining pulse rates, the individual may become dizzy—or even faint—when he suddenly changes from a reclining to a standing position.

Check your pulse occasionally by placing the finger tips of your right hand over the thumbside of the inside portion of your left wrist. If your resting pulse rate has not decreased after several weeks of exercising, see your doctor for a checkup. If everything is OK, try increasing the amount of exercise you do.

The average pulse rate while sitting is about 72 beats per minute. When you're in good condition, it will drop to 65 or less. A minister who had a resting pulse rate of 90 beats per minute lost 25 pounds of fat and reduced his heart rate to 60 by following a progressive program of walking and jogging. The weight loss greatly reduced the workload on his heart, and his circulation improved so much that many of his chronic aches and pains disappeared.

"Since I started exercising," he said, "I sleep better and I have a lot more endurance. When my pulse rate began to drop, I began to feel younger and more energetic."

If your pulse rate is consistently higher than it should be, you may be speeding along the road to premature old age and an early death. If you can keep your pulse rate low by conditioning your muscles and your heart, however, you can delay the aging process and build up a reserve for many extra years of precious life.

SUMMARY

1. Trim all fat from the meat you eat and cut down on the total amount of fat in your diet. This will prevent a build-up of fat in your blood and in your tissues.

2. Eliminate all sugar and refined foods from your diet and eat such low-fat foods as chicken, fish, liver, cottage cheese, whole grain cereals, fruits, and vegetables. Drink skim milk.

3. Do not use products containing hydrogenated vegetable oil, lard, or chemical preservatives.

4. Use vegetable oil on your salads and supplement your diet with lecithin. This will emulsify the hard fat in your blood so that it won't clog your arteries.

5. Brewer's yeast will supply important B vitamins that the body needs to produce its own lecithin.

6. Two tablespoons of wheat germ oil each day will supply Vitamin E and the essential fatty acids, both of which are important in preventing atherosclerosis or hardened arteries.

7. Coffee and cigarettes constrict blood vessels, speed the heart rate, and increase the amount of fat and cholesterol in the blood. Alcohol destroys important B vitamins and interferes with the liver's production of lecithin.

8. Regular exercise, performed at least twice a week, will strengthen your heart, lower your resting pulse rate, widen your coronary arteries, and reduce the amount of fat and cholesterol in your blood.

9. Unrelieved nervous tension can deprive the heart of adequate blood by constricting the coronary arteries and raising blood fat.

10. Rest, recreation, and emotional tranquility are just as important to good health as proper diet and regular exercise.

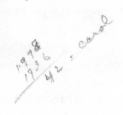

10

How to Keep Your Spine Youthful and Flexible for Better Health

There are 26 vertebrae in the normal spine. Including the rib joints and discs, there are about 135 joints that allow you to bend, breathe, and move about. Most of us take our flexibility for granted until a strain or injury causes paralyzing pain. When old age begins to stiffen the joints of the spine, the individual is constantly reminded of his "decrepit condition."

It's bad enough not to be able to do all the things you used to do when you were younger, but worse things can happen if your spine stiffens from inactivity. Your general health, for example, will be adversely affected, and the harm that results may speed the aging process.

There are many young people who have a stiff spine that could be loosened with manipulation or exercise. So no matter what your age might be, you can benefit from the spinal adjusting techniques described in this chapter. With a flexible spine and properly aligned vertebrae, you'll have a better chance of being the youthful, vigorous person you want to be.

160

GOOD BODY MECHANICS AND A FLEXIBLE SPINE CAN
PREVENT DISEASE AND DELAY THE AGING PROCESS

The vertebral column houses the spinal cord, which is literally an extension of the brain. And all along the way nerve trunks branch out from the cord and pass between the vertebrae to supply muscles, skin, and other tissues with the electrical energy that gives them life. Some of the nerve centers supplying the heart, blood vessels, and other organs rest against the vertebrae in a chain that runs up and down both sides of the spinal column.

When your spine is healthy and flexible, there is plenty of room between the vertebrae for the nerve trunks. When it stiffens from disease or lack of exercise, however, compression of discs and thickening of ligaments and joints crowd the nerves and irritate important nerve centers. If one of the spinal nerves is pinched or irritated, pain or numbness may radiate into an arm or a leg. The overall effect of a stiff spine, however, may be a painless progression of the aging process. Circulatory interference and nerve irritation can cause a great variety of symptoms. Organs may not function efficiently. Tight muscles may create harmful tension that will prevent healthful relaxation and restful sleep. Strained posture and sore joints may trigger muscle spasm, headaches, and other aches and pains.

According to Joel E. Goldthwait, M.D., in his book *Body Mechanics in Health and Disease* (J.B. Lippincott Company, Philadelphia, 1952), sagging of the spine, abdomen, and rib cage in chronic postural distortions can cause such diseases as arthritis, diabetes, heart strain, high blood pressure, stomach ulcers, kidney stones, psoriasis, bursitis, arteriosclerosis, hernia, varicose veins, and even cancer by obstructing circulation and placing pressure on joints, nerves, and organs. Diabetes, for example, might be caused by pressure placed upon the pancreas by a curved spine and congested abdominal organs. Circulatory congestion in the liver might cause heart strain.

Pressure upon the adrenal glands might trigger a hormone imbalance that could cause skin disease, and so on. So it's very important to have good posture supported by a straight, healthy spine and well-toned muscles.

BUILDING YOUTHFUL POSTURE

Good posture is essential to good spinal health. If you allow your spine to sag and slump most of the day, your vertebrae will eventually change their shape so that your spine will become permanently distorted. Once this happens, the pull of gravity on the unbalanced spine will tend to increase the distortion. Furthermore, shortening of muscles and ligaments on one side of the curved spine will make it very difficult to loosen your vertebrae adequately.

How to Stand

Always remember to *stand tall.* Maintain your maximum height with a straight spine. But don't try too hard. If your posture is not easy and relaxed, you won't be able to maintain it for very long.

Lift your chest a little. Hold your abdomen in just enough to keep it from bulging. Keep your toes pointed straight ahead, with most of your weight supported on the outside edges of the soles of your feet. (See Figure 10-1.)

How to Sit

When you sit in a chair, sit upright with a slight arch in your lower back. On long automobile trips, you can place a folded towel in the small of your back to help you maintain a relaxed sitting posture.

When you use a hard straight-backed chair, it should be just high enough to let both feet rest on the floor with only a small amount of pressure on the back of your thighs. When the chair is too high, the edge of seat may place damaging pressure on important nerves just above and behind your knees.

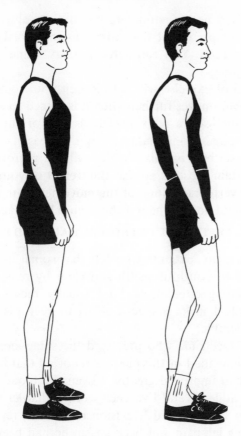

Figure 10-1. *Good posture builds good health. Bad posture places pressure on nerves and organs.*

HOW TO ADJUST YOUR SPINE WHILE YOU RELAX YOUR MUSCLES

If you'd like to strengthen the muscles in your back, you'll find a complete course of barbell and freehand exercises in my book *Backache: Home Treatment and Prevention* (Parker Publishing Company, West Nyack, New York). In the meantime, you can loosen and stretch your spine, align your vertebrae, free nerves, stimulate circulation, and relax muscles with no more effort than turning over in bed or hanging from a tree limb. You can actually *relax* while you adjust your own spine.

Any kind of exercise will help loosen your spine. A spinal joint, however, moves further when it is forced to move while the back muscles are relaxed. This is one of the secrets of successful spinal manipulation. For this reason, the special postures described in this chapter will be performed while relaxing certain muscles, so that the weight of your body will move your vertebrae. None of the movements are dangerous, but you should not do them if they cause back pain.

FEEL BETTER WITH A PROPERLY ALIGNED SPINE

I've had many patients who felt that spinal manipulation contributed to youthful health and vigor by releasing nerves and stimulating circulation. So I usually recommend that each individual make a special effort to keep his own spine loose and flexible.

An auto mechanic who practiced the spine-loosening postures recommended in this chapter reported that his stomach condition had improved greatly. "Even my blood pressure is down," he added, "and I've been working harder than ever."

Jonathan R., a retired television repairman, reported that the recurring leg pain and back spasm he had been suffering from for years did not return after practicing the special postures for only two weeks. "It might be my imagination," he said, "but I believe my circulation has improved, and I feel better all over."

It wasn't Jonathan's imagination that he was feeling better. When you loosen a stiff spine, an improvement in body mechanics can have a beneficial effect on every structure in the body.

STIFF HIPS CAN GIVE YOU A STIFF SPINE

Most people will attempt to test the flexibility of their

spine by bending over to touch their toes. What they're really testing, however, is hip flexibility, which is actually a measure of the tightness of the hamstring muscles on the back of the thighs. In other words, when you bend forward with straight legs, the amount of bending that takes place in your hips is limited by the pull of muscles that attach to the back of your pelvis. Since tightness in the hamstrings is usually a sign of loss of youthful flexibility, the spine may also be stiff. So one of the first things you have to do to regain your flexibility is to stretch your hamstrings.

Because of the danger of low-back strain or disc injury in toe-touching exercises, you shouldn't try to touch your toes while standing erect. Instead, you can stretch your hamstrings in a relaxed sitting position.

Sit Down and Stretch Your Hamstrings

Sit on the floor with your feet together and your legs locked out straight. Lean forward as far as you can while lightly pulling on your legs with your hands. Don't do the exercise rapidly or forcefully. Stop the forced flexion when the stretch on the back of your legs begins to be a little painful. (See Figure 10-2.)

Exhale while bending forward. Keep your back and abdominal muscles *relaxed* while you pull with your arms.

LOOSENING THE LOWER SPINE

The spinal cord ends at the level of the 2nd lumbar vertebra, which is just above the beltline. There are, however, plenty of nerves that reach down from the spinal cord to pass out from between the lumbar vertebrae. Many of them supply important pelvic structures along with the thighs and legs.

Since the lumbar spine is usually the first part of the back to stiffen from age or inactivity, you should begin early to make a special effort to keep it flexible if you want to avoid

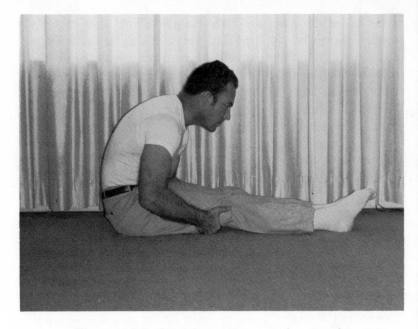

Figure 10-2 *Stretching the muscles on the back of the thighs helps to restore youthful flexibility.*

"old age backache" caused by compression of discs and nerves.

A 60-year-old woman who complained of constipation, backache, and leg ache reported complete relief from all these disturbances after practicing the next two loosening exercises. "I adjust my own spine, " she says, "and the results have been gratifying."

It has been my observation that constipation frequently accompanies severe or chronic backache. The reason for this, I believe, is that the nerve supply to the colon is disturbed by the pain and spasm of lumbar nerves and muscles. In these cases, the constipation disappears when the back trouble is corrected. Chronic constipation can, of course, *cause* backache, so be sure to read Chapter 5 for tips on how to establish youthful regularity.

The Kneeling Back Arch

Get down on your hands and knees. Drop your head down while arching your back up as high as you can. Then lift your head while letting your spine sag. *Relax* the muscles of your back and abdomen in the sagging position so that your spine will be pulled down by the weight of your abdomen. Alternately arch your back up and then let it sag. (See Figures 10-3 and 10-4.)

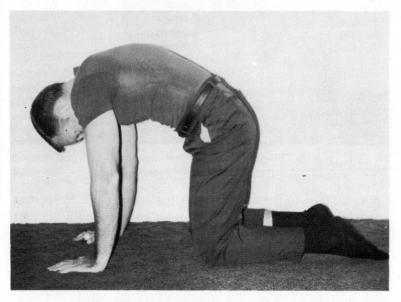

Figure 10-3 *Arching your back upward loosens spinal joints and releases nerves.*

The Lying Twist for the Lower Spine

Lie flat on your back with your arms at your sides and your thighs and legs flexed. In other words, bend your hips and your knees and lift your feet off the floor. Hold your legs together in this bent position and drop them first to one

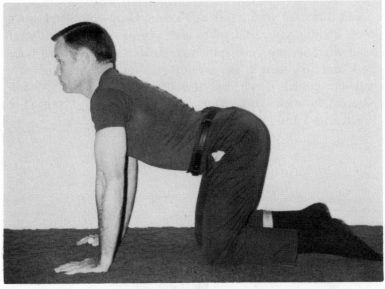

Figure 10-4 *Arching your back downward loosens spinal joints and expands discs.*

side and then to the other by twisting at the waist. Keep your upper back flat on the floor in order to increase the amount of rotation in your lower spine. (See Figure 10-5.)

Each time you lower your legs to the floor, *relax* your abdominal and back muscles for a couple of seconds at the completion of the movement so that the weight of your legs will force some additional rotation of the vertebrae.

A welder I know uses this exercise to unlock a recurring "kink" in his lower back. "It also seems to relieve the arthritic stiffness in my spine," he added.

THE CARPET-ROLL ADJUSTMENT FOR THE UPPER SPINE

As we grow older, there is a tendency for the upper back to sag. Thinning of the discs and softening of the vertebrae may allow the pull of gravity to telescope the dorsal spine

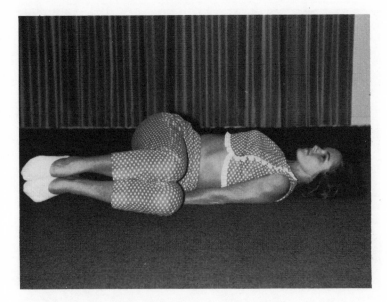

Figure 10-5 *The lying twist will adjust and align the lumbar vertebrae.*

into a hump-back curvature. You can prevent this, however, by using the carpet-roll adjustment two or three times a week.

Roll up a piece of carpet padding as tightly as you can and tie it on each end with a piece of string. Place the roll on the floor and lie back over it so that it presses into the most prominent part of your upper back. Place your hands behind your head and *relax* so that the weight of your body will straighten your spine and adjust your vertebrae. (See Figure 10-6.)

There may be times when this simple adjustment will relieve chest pain as well as back pain. Robert R., for example, a 45-year-old dairy farmer, had been complaining of chest pain for several months. Since the pain was on the left side of his chest, he had his heart examined by a cardiologist.

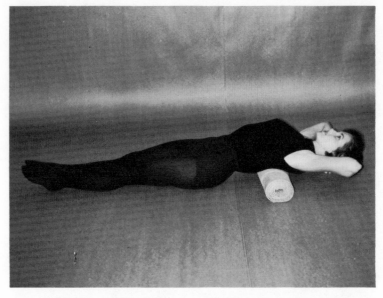

Figure 10-6 *A carpet roll placed under the upper back will adjust the dorsal vertebrae.*

The tests were negative. When he tried the carpet-roll treatment, his back "popped" and the pain disappeared. What had appeared to be a heart pain was simply a nerve pain that was radiating into his chest from a stiff spinal joint.

A Sacroiliac Adjustment

Place the roll under your hips and lie relaxed for a few seconds. This will force your sacroiliac joints into proper position and stretch your hip flexors. Remove the roll when you begin to feel a little pain or discomfort. (See Figure 10-7.)

THE LEANING SIDE BEND TO STRETCH YOUR BACK MUSCLES

Stand about one foot away from a wall and at right angles to it. Then lean against the wall with your hip.

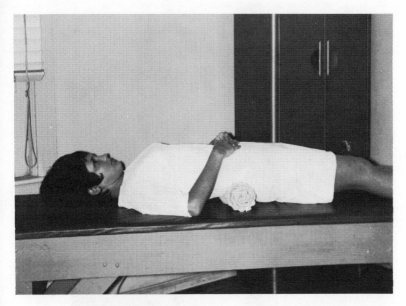

Figure 10-7 *A carpet roll under the hips will adjust the sacroiliac joints.*

Bend your upper body away from the wall so that your spine curves to one side. Keep your knees locked out straight and let your arms hang relaxed. *Relax* the muscles of your trunk as much as possible so that the weight of your upper body will stretch the thigh and back muscles on the side of your body next to the wall. (See Figure 10-8.)

Maintain the leaning posture for two or three seconds or until the pull on your spine becomes a little uncomfortable.

One of my patients who complained of backache and aching hips that defied diagnosis and treatment obtained complete relief with this simple exercise. Stretching of tight bands of connective tissue on the outside of her thighs simply relieved an abnormal pull on her hips and her spine.

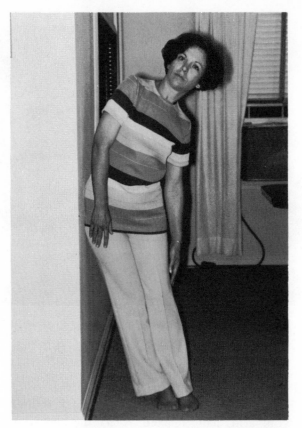

Figure 10-8 *The leaning side bend stretches muscles on one side of the body.*

HOW TO USE A SLANT BOARD TO STRETCH YOUR SPINE

One of the best and most comfortable ways to stretch your entire spine and its muscles is to lie down on a slant board with your feet anchored at the high end of the board. The steeper the incline of the board, the greater the pull on your spine. Discs will expand, and pressure on joints and nerves will be relieved. Your body will become vibrantly alive with a new flow of blood and nerve impulses.

Prop the board (a plank that's about one inch thick, 12 inches wide, and seven feet long) up on a table or some other fairly high surface. Secure your feet with a strap and lie on the board perfectly relaxed. You'll be able to feel the pull on your spine.

I once recommended the slant board for an overweight waitress who complained of backache, abdominal pains, leg numbness, dizziness, and a variety of other symptoms of unknown origin. Lying on the board for about ten minutes a couple of times each day relieved *all* of these complaints, and it did so when a half-dozen other treatments had no effect at all. Reversing the effects of gravity simply relieved postural strains and removed pressure on nerves, blood vessels, and organs. Everyone should lie down on a slant board occasionally. The effects might be helpful in reversing the aging process.

It might also be a good idea to hang from a chinning bar or a tree limb occasionally. Just grip the bar with both hands and hang as relaxed as you can for a few seconds.

BREATHE TO STRETCH YOUR RIB CAGE

Any exercise that forces expansion of your rib cage will help you keep a straight spine. Many of the muscles used in lifting the ribs also support the spine. If you allow your rib cage to sink and flatten, your upper spine might sag into a hump, squeezing your heart and lungs and creating a stiff back.

You can stretch your rib cage and lift your vertebrae effectively with a simple isometric exercise that takes only a few seconds to perform.

Lie down on the floor, reach back over your head with straight arms, and hook both hands under the bottom edge of a heavy sofa or cedar chest. Then inhale deeply while exerting a little upward pressure with your hands. Be sure to keep your abdominal muscles *relaxed* so that the muscles in your chest and upper back can lift your ribs while you expand your lungs. (If you do this exercise, you don't have to do the "isometric chest expander" described in Chapter 7.)

Women as well as men can use this exercise to improve their physical appearance by lifting up a sagging chest. (See Figure 10-9.)

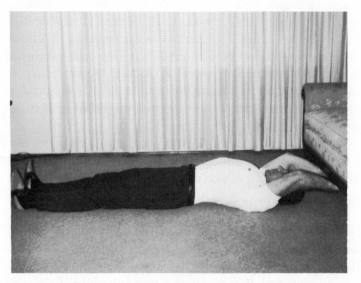

Figure 10-9 *Inhaling deeply while performing the isometric sofa lift will expand the lungs and stretch the rib cage.*

TWO SPECIAL EXERCISES TO TONE UP SUPPORTING MUSCLES

If you'd like to take a small amount of exercise to tone up the muscles supporting your spine, there are two very simple and basic exercises that you can do in bed or on the floor.

The Spinal Bridge

Lie on your back with your knees bent and both feet flat

on the floor. Rest your hands on your abdomen and lift your back from the floor so that your weight is supported on your feet and your shoulders. Do 12 to 20 repetitions. You can make the exercise a little harder and more effective by holding a sand bag on your abdomen. Ten or 15 pounds should be adequate. (See Figure 10-10.)

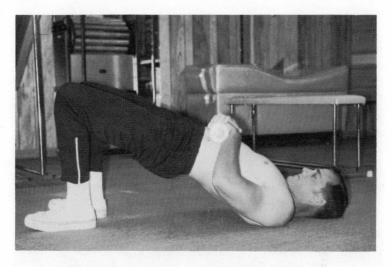

Figure 10-10 *The spinal bridge strengthens back muscles without placing a strain on joints and discs.*

This exercise will activate hip and thigh muscles as well as the long spina erecta muscles running up and down each side of your spine.

The Bent-Knee Leg Raise

The muscles supporting the front of the spine are just as important as those in back. Therefore, you should include an exercise that will tone up your abdominal muscles and your hip flexors. You can do this easily with bent-knee leg raises.

Lie on your back with your knees slightly bent, feet together, and both heels on the floor. Hold your knees in a bent position and raise both legs together until your feet are directly over your abdomen. Keep your arms alongside your body so that you can exert a balancing counter pressure with your hands. Do 12 to 15 repetitions. (See Figure 10-11.)

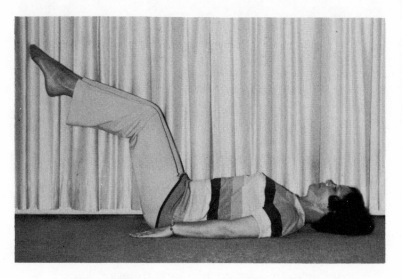

Figure 10-11 *The knees should be kept bent during leg raises.*

A STIMULATING BACK TREATMENT

Everyone likes a good back rub. You can combine all the pleasures of back massage with a stimulating circulatory and nerve treatment by following a simple routine that employs moist heat, massage, and a small hand vibrator.

Wring out a couple of towels in hot water and apply them up and down the length of the spine.

When the towels have cooled, remove them and cover the back with a generous amount of oil or cream.

Cup one hand over the ridge of muscle on one side of the spine and tuck a rubber vibrator cup under the thumb and first finger of that hand. Then stroke the muscle *from bottom to top* by moving the hand and the vibrator together. The pressure of the massaging hand will push blood through the muscle, while the vibrator will stimulate nerves. (See Figure 10-12.)

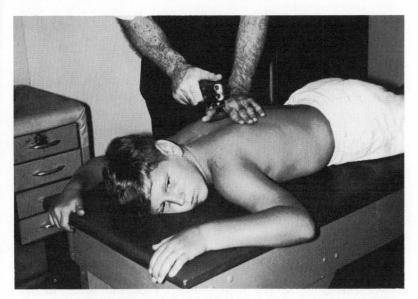

Figure 10-12 *Combining massage and vibration will stimulate nerves and increase the circulation of blood.*

Use an alcohol rub to remove the oil and cool the skin. If you'd like to conclude the treatment with a really potent stimulant, try rubbing the spine very briefly with an ice cube. This will charge the nerves with youthful energy that will radiate into all the organs of the body.

SUMMARY

1. Your spine is the lifeline of your body. It houses the spinal cord and distributes nerves to every portion of your body.

2. Keeping your spine flexible will prevent irritation of nerves; keeping it straight will prevent compression of organs.

3. In practicing good posture, remember to *stand tall,* point your toes nearly straight ahead, and support your weight on the outside edges of the soles of your feet.

4. Practice the spine-loosening postures described in this chapter at least once a week.

5. Do not attempt to loosen your spine by touching your toes in a standing position.

6. Expanding your rib cage and lifting your chest with breathing exercises will help prevent sagging of your chest and upper spine.

7. There are two simple exercises—described in this chapter—that will tone up the muscles supporting your spine.

8. Moist heat applications over the spine, followed by back massage with a hand vibrator, will stimulate nerves and blood vessels that pass between the vertebrae.

9. Rubbing the spine with an ice cube following a moist heat application is an effective nerve stimulant for robust persons.

10. Try to hang from a tree limb or a chinning bar occasionally to stretch your muscles and your spine—or lie relaxed on a steep slant board.

11

How to Keep Your Body Youthful, Slim, and Attractive

Most of the popular books on diet and exercise are so complicated and lengthy that the average person cannot begin to make practical use of them. In this chapter, I have outlined a simple diet and exercise plan that anyone can follow. And the program is so effective that you won't need any additional instructions in building the kind of youthful, slim body that everyone admires so much.

If you normally tend to be overweight, you may have to work a little harder than the average person to keep your body attractive. You can rest assured, however, that your efforts will be well rewarded. Just remember that you can't be truly youthful and vigorous if your body is fat and flabby.

Too much fat can, in fact, kill you! So even if you don't care how you look, you shouldn't carry around any more fat than necessary if you want to live out your allotted life span. *If you can pinch up more than a half-inch thickness of fat over your abdomen, you have too much flab.*

Homer C. was one of those misinformed persons who didn't worry about his physical appearance—until he began to fear for his life. "I don't care how I look," he once said when I suggested that he reduce his body weight and tone up his muscles. "I'm not a vain egoist. Besides, my wife is just as fat as I am."

Several months later, Homer began to complain of chest pains, and he had difficulty breathing. When a heart specialist told him that fat was crowding his heart and lungs, he finally agreed to reduce. The threat of death was enough to convince him that he had to do something about his weight.

Several months after making a few simple changes in his way of life, Homer was 40 pounds lighter and still losing. "I feel great," he said. "My chest pain is gone and I can breathe all right. I no longer feel that uncomfortable pressure in my abdomen when I lie down or sit down. My wife is following the same program, and she's looking better every day. In fact, her honeymoon beauty is busting out all over. I wish we had taken your advice years ago."

Carolyn R., a 37-year-old divorcee who wanted to remarry, regained her youthful figure—and vigor—by eating the type of food recommended in this chapter. "I never knew that weight reducing could be so easy," she said after following the diet plan for a few months. "I always thought you had to starve yourself, or at least count your calories. My friends are telling me how good I look . . . and I met the nicest man the other day."

You can follow the same diet and exercise program that Homer and Carolyn followed, and with equally good results. Best of all, *you won't have to go hungry a single day.*

THE DANGERS OF OVERWEIGHT

Everybody wants to look good and be physically attractive. That's reason enough to avoid gaining excessive weight. The health benefits, however, are even more important. Overweight contributes to the development of heart disease, hardened arteries, diabetes, strokes, high blood pressure, arthritis, and other disorders that cause premature aging if not an early death.

It's well known that obesity shortens life. Each pound of excess fat overworks the heart with miles of surplus blood vessels. The added burden on muscles, joints, and ligaments causes a multitude of aches and pains. Wounds heal slowly, and recovery from surgery is prolonged.

Overweight can also wreck your sex life. If your body is distorted by bulging, flabby fat, the sight of it may "turn off" your mate—or you may find the physical side of sexual activity difficult and fatiguing. With a firm youthful body, however, you can be attractive and active for as long as you live, even if you live to be 100. (See Figure 11-1.)

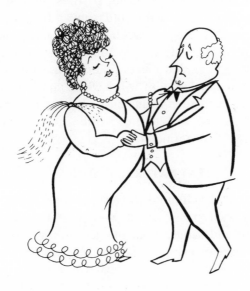

Figure 11-1 *Overweight can ruin your love life as well as cause premature aging.*

George Bernard Shaw once said that "youth is wasted on the young." If you put into effect what you learn in all the chapters of this book, you won't lose your youthfulness before you are too old to appreciate it. It's especially important that you pay attention to what you eat.

BEGIN BY ELIMINATING HIGH-CALORIE FOODS

Most people who are overweight are simply eating too many refined or processed foods that contain white sugar or white flour—or both. Since refined sugar and flour are highly concentrated carbohydrates, they contribute far too many calories in the diet of the average person.

If you're overweight, you should *eliminate all foods containing white sugar or white flour.* This means that shouldn't eat candy, white bread, pastries, pies, cake, spaghetti, commercial ice cream, and similar foods. And you shouldn't drink beverages that have been sweetened with sugar. One piece of candy or a spoonful of sugar will supply more calories than several pieces of fresh, nutritious fruit. If you eat candy each day, you will have to cut down on more wholesome foods to keep from consuming too many calories. No one can afford to sacrifice fruits and vegetables for commercial sweets or refined foods.

EAT NATURAL FOODS

When your diet is limited to fresh, natural foods that are not prepared with grease or oil, you should be able to fill your stomach and satisfy your hunger without taking in an excessive number of calories. You won't even have to count your calories or keep a record of what you eat.

Turn back to Chapter 4 and review the material on how to plan and prepare a balanced meal. Then select your foods from lean meat, fish, chicken, eggs, skim milk, cottage cheese, fruits, vegetables, and whole grain cereals and breads. Eat *fresh* foods that have not been preserved with chemical additives.

Eat Plenty of Fish and Chicken

Fish and chicken are high in protein and low in fat. When they are baked or broiled, you can eat just about all you want. You should, however, peel the skin from chicken to eliminate surface fat.

Egg yolk is fairly rich in fat, so you probably should not eat more than a couple of eggs each day if you're eating meat and drinking whole milk. I doubt that anyone could get fat eating boiled eggs, but the cholesterol content of egg yolk may contribute to the development of atherosclerosis or hardened arteries.

Drink Skim Milk or Vegetable Juice

You should always try to drink a little skim milk or fruit or vegetable juice with your meals. In addition to supplying essential food elements, these beverages help to satisfy the appetite by filling the stomach.

Fruit juice contains some sugar, but vegetable juices are relatively sugar free. Tomato juice is a good breakfast beverage for overweight persons, and it's rich in youth-building Vitamin C.

Vegetables Won't Make You Fat

As a rule, you don't have to worry about getting too many calories from vegetables. Rutabagas, cabbage, squash, asparagus, turnips, collards, spinach, string beans, tomatoes, okra, and other readily available *fresh* vegetables can be served generously. If you are overweight, however, you may have to eat less of such starchy vegetables as peas and potatoes.

If you eat a variety of vegetables in a balanced diet, it's not likely that you will overeat or take in too many calories. When the appetite is satisfied with fresh, natural foods, a balance between bulk (cellulose) and calories provides a built-in protection against a build-up of body fat.

Visit the grocery store each day and shop for fresh, crispy

vegetables. Try them all. Properly prepared without grease or oil, almost any vegetable is a low calorie source of youth-building vitamins and minerals. Frozen vegetables are all right if they are properly packaged and cared for. But whenever possible, select fresh vegetables that are "in season" so that you will get more taste as well as food value for your money.

Load Up on Salads

Fresh, raw vegetable salads are also great for providing nutritious, low-calorie bulk and satisfying the appetite. A big bowl of lettuce and tomatoes sprinkled with string beans, bean sprouts, diced beets, cottage cheese, wheat germ, or some other low-calorie food, for example, can provide a tasty and refreshing dish. Any raw vegetable that suits your palate can be shredded and mixed into a salad.

A few drops of vinegar or lemon juice can replace oily salad dressings.

Eat Sweets Provided by Nature

Although you shouldn't eat commercial sweets that contain refined sugar, you can benefit from sweets provided by nature. Fresh or dried fruits, for example, are loaded with vitamins and minerals, and they're infinitely more delicious than candy or ice cream.

A banana or half an apple with a few dates or a handful of raisins makes a nourishing and satisfying dessert. A little honey mixed with peanut butter and spread over a graham cracker will satisfy anyone's craving for something sweet.

You should absolutely refuse to eat "diet foods" and beverages that have been artificially sweetened. There is now some reason to believe that chemical sweeteners may contribute to the development of cancer and other diseases.

HOW A COLLEGE TEACHER LOST 46 POUNDS

Arnold B., a college teacher who suffered from "bad feet"

and high blood pressure, relieved both of these complaints by reducing his weight from 226 pounds to 180 pounds. Although he ate a variety of fresh, natural foods, his diet was composed primarily of the following foods:

For breakfast, Arnold had whole wheat cereal with skim milk (sweetened with honey or raisins), a piece of fresh fruit, a scrambled egg, and a glass of tomato juice.

Dinner consisted of baked chicken or fish, two fresh vegetables cooked in waterless cookware, a slice of home-made whole wheat bread, and a glass of fruit juice.

Supper was made up of small servings of dinner leftovers, supplemented by a bowl of raw vegetable salad and a glass of skim milk. If he still felt hungry, he had a piece of fresh or dried fruit with a cup of wheat germ cereal.

"I believe I actually eat *more* than I used to," Arnold said after losing several pounds. "But by cutting out processed foods and taking a little exercise, I've been able to lose weight without starving myself. And all those vitamins and minerals I've been getting have made me look and feel much younger than my 50 years."

HOW TO COUNT YOUR CALORIES

If you restrict your diet to the type of low-calorie foods recommended in this chapter and then take a small amount of regular exercise, you can trim down and tone up without depriving your stomach. But if you'd like to count your calories so that you can include measured portions of high-calorie foods, you can do so by using a simple formula. It's important to remember, however, that if you eat candy, commercial ice cream, and other refined sweets, or drink beer or sugar-sweetened beverages, you will have to make a drastic cut in the amount of food you eat. A few tablespoons of sugar can replace all the fruits and vegetables you would need to meet your calorie requirements in a balanced diet, but pure sugar won't provide the vitamins and minerals you need to be youthful and vigorous. I would much rather "fill up" on lean meat, fruits, and vegetables than count my calories in a skimpy meal that includes pie and ice cream.

Maintaining Body Weight with 15 Calories per Pound

Nutritional scientists tell us that we need about 15 calories per pound of body weight each day to keep from losing or gaining weight. A person weighing 200 pounds, for example, would need about 3,000 calories daily (200 x 15 = 3,000) to maintain that weight. If you take in more calories than you need, you gain weight, and vice versa.

Each pound of fat your body stores contains about 3,500 calories. This means that if you want to lose a pound of fat each week, you must make sure that the total number of calories you take in each day is 500 less than you need to maintain your existing weight. Then, when your body is as lean as you want it to be, you can stop the progressive reduction in calories and just concentrate on maintaining your weight.

You can pick up a calorie chart in a drug store or at your local library to help you "measure" the foods you eat.

It's never a good idea to attempt to lose more than a couple of pounds a week. "Crash diets" that starve your body so that it is forced to get most of its fuel from stored fat can be dangerous. Excessive combustion of fat can cause illness by overloading the body with toxins.

Since fatty tissue increases your need for certain vitamins and minerals, your food intake must be gradually and progressively reduced as the fat disappears. Otherwise, there may not be enough calcium, Vitamin C, and other youth-building elements to supply essential tissues and organs along with the parasitic fat cells.

"Crash diets," says Dr. Thomas Cureton of the University of Illinois, "lower the resistance and leave the individual prone to disease, fatigue, unnatural aging, and other harmful effects."

BEWARE OF FAD DIETS

A good reducing diet *must* contain a small amount of carbohydrate, so that your body won't be forced to burn more than an optimum amount of body fat to meet your daily energy requirement. You should *never* go on a "starvation diet," or a diet that calls for strict use of a single food or beverage. No one should ever totally eliminate fruits, vegetables, and milk. Remember what you learned in Chapter 4 about the importance of certain vitamins and minerals in building youthful health and vigor. Your bowels must also have cellulose to function properly, and you cannot get this from meat or from hard boiled eggs (see Chapter 5).

Some fad diets recommend that you take vitamin pills to make up for the deficiencies in such diets. It's important to remember, however, that natural foods may contain undiscovered vitamins, minerals, and enzymes that cannot be found in a bottle. For this reason, every diet—even a reducing diet—must be made up of a balanced variety of all types of foods.

The only way to get rid of excess body fat permanently is to develop good eating habits and then stick with them for the rest of your life. If you eat properly, your daily diet can also be your reducing diet. You won't ever have to starve yourself with a "crash diet" that does more harm than good.

Ideally speaking, *you should not gain any weight at all after age 25.*

PREVENT OVERWEIGHT AND TONE YOUR MUSCLES WITH EXERCISE

There are some nutritionists, including Dr. Jean Mayer of Harvard University, who maintain that *inactivity or lack or exercise is the biggest cause of overweight.* There is no doubt that most people are eating too much fattening food, but many of them would not be overweight if they were more active.

When your body metabolism is stimulated by even a small amount of regular exercise, you can eat considerably more of your favorite fattening foods without gaining weight. When you are completely sedentary, however, it's almost impossible to avoid building up a little flab, even on the most restricted diet. Furthermore, muscles that are not exercised will sag under the weight of accumulating fat, causing hideous distortion of the body.

The human body wasn't designed for a completely sedentary life—and it shouldn't be starved by "crash diets." So if you want to be truly youthful and vigorous, and if you want to *look* good, you will have to take a little exercise as well as eat properly. This doesn't mean that you have to torture yourself by running ten miles or by doing hundreds of push-ups. There are many ways to get the exercise you need through recreational activity.

How to Enjoy Your Exercise

For any exercise to be effective, it must be done regularly. Few people, however, will continue any form of exercise they do not enjoy. For this reason, it's important that your exercise be recreational in nature. Handball, volleyball, swimming, tennis, basketball, or bicycle riding, for example, can offer adequate fun-type exercise for most people. Any sport or athletic activity that involves use of the legs is great for burning calories.

If you eat properly and you're not already overweight, simply walking, working in the yard, or playing golf will stimulate your body metabolism enough to prevent an abnormal accumulation of body fat.

The important thing is to stay active. Don't spend all of your spare time eating snacks and watching television. No matter how busy you think you are, make sure that you indulge in some type of physical activity that you enjoy doing at least every other day—preferably every day.

Walk to the grocery store whenever possible. Take every opportunity you get to walk along a seashore or through a forest. Even a walk through the neighborhood can be entertaining. I particularly enjoy riding a bicycle through residential areas that I do not often get a chance to visit. You would be surprised at the things you see and the people you meet on such a journey.

Stay Active with a Hobby

A hobby that calls for physical activity can keep you lean and fit. Golf, for example, will do more for your body than chess or cards. Hiking or camping has more to offer than shooting clay pigeons or making ceramics. Swimming can be more fun than fishing—and it's certainly more strenuous. Getting outdoors and exposing your skin to sun, air, and water is a youth-building tonic that you cannot afford to be without.

Whatever type of exercise you do, you'll do more than enough if you really enjoy doing it. I've seen middle-aged men play handball until they were nearly exhausted—and enjoy every minute of it. Many people who play volleyball on the beach for hours at a time could not be persuaded to do a single push-up at home. I know a 60-year-old insurance salesman who jumps rope. He spends hours developing skills in the use of a rope, and he puts on a beautiful performance. You, too, can enjoy the right kind of exercise, and you can stay youthfully slim doing it.

THE FALLACY OF SPOT REDUICNG

You don't have to take a special exercise to reduce a certain portion of your body. Fat deposits represent stored calories, and no matter where they are in your body, they can be burned off with any endurance-type exercise that requires the use of your legs. It's simply a matter of burning more calories each day than you take in. If you eat properly, you can burn body fat with only a small amount of exercise.

Be guided by the effects of the food you eat and the exercise you take. If you find weight reduction inadequate or too slow, you can either cut down on the amount of food you eat or you can increase the amount of exercise you do—or both.

Don't be taken in by mechanical reducing machines that are supposed to remove fat by rolling it away or vibrating it off. The only way you can get rid of body fat is to burn it as energy.

SUMMARY

1. In addition to making you look bad, too much body fat can shorten your life and contribute to the development of a number of diseases.

2. The first rule of successful dieting in weight reduction is to eliminate *all* foods containing white sugar and white flour.

3. Avoid refined or processed foods and eat fresh, natural foods that have not been prepared with grease or oil.

4. Basically, a balanced reducing diet should be made up of foods selected from lean meat, fish, chicken, eggs, skim milk, cottage cheese, fresh fruits, fresh vegetables, and whole grain breads and cereals.

5. Drink fruit juice for breakfast, vegetable juice at dinner, and skim milk at supper.

6. Eat salads containing a variety of raw, edible vegetables. Use vinegar or lemon juice rather than oily salad dressings.

7. Satisfy your sweet tooth with fresh or dried fruits.

8. If you take a little regular exercise and eat the type of foods recommended in this chapter, you should be able to control your body weight with no trouble at all.

9. If you'd like to calculate your intake of calories,

remember that it takes about 15 calories per pound of body weight to maintain your *existing* weight.

10. You must be *active* to be truly lean and vigorous. Select a form of exercise that you enjoy doing—something that you can do for the rest of your life.

12

How to Cultivate a Smooth, Youthful Skin at Any Age

The skin is a very important organ. In addition to pro-viding beauty for the eye and pleasure for the touch, the cutaneous sac in which we live helps to regulate body temperature and prevent disease. It eliminates waste and provides us with warning sensations of pain. It even absorbs a certain amount of oxygen. Many diseases of the body are reflected by the appearance of the skin, making it easier for your doctor to diagnose your illnesses.

There are many types of skin disease, all of which must be treated by a doctor. But good nutrition, which plays an important role in building attractive skin, can also *prevent* skin disease. A deficiency in Vitamin A, for example, reduces the skin's ability to resist infection by germs, fungus, and parasites. Lack of adequate Vitamin B causes pellagra, a horrible-looking skin disease. When there is not enough Vitamin C in the diet, tissue cells fall apart and capillaries break and bleed.

Iron gives the skin its pleasant, pink glow. Vitamin F (the unsaturated fatty acids) keeps it soft and pliable and velvety.

The skin itself is made from protein, which is best supplied by foods of animal origin. There are many minerals, such as iodine, that help to keep the skin healthy and attractive.

Obviously, the first thing you must do to cultivate a healthy skin is to eat properly. So be sure to study the material in Chapter 4. Although your skin is on the outside, it must be fed from the inside.

There are also certain special procedures that you must carry out in caring for the *surface* of your skin if you want to be physically attractive and youthful in appearance.

CASE HISTORIES OF BETTY, CARLOS, AND ROBERTA

When I was a student in college, I knew a lovely and popular young lady, Betty J., who stayed fit and trim by taking regular exercise. She spent long hours in the sun each day and had acquired a beautiful, dark tan. When I saw her again 20 years later, she was still physically fit and she still had a dark tan. Her skin was thick and wrinkled, however, and her face was heavily coated with make-up to conceal acne-like eruptions on her chin, She looked very much like an old woman trying to look young. No one believed that she was only 38 years of age. Her *skin* made her look 20 years older than she really was.

Carlos C. was a 28-year-old bachelor who had been engaged to the same girl for two years. He wanted to get married, but a skin problem had forced him to postpone the marriage on two different occasions. "I've got a bad skin infection on my feet and around my groin," he said, "and I just can't expose my girl to that on our wedding night. Besides, it might be contagious."

The skin problems of both Betty and Carlos could easily have been prevented. All that would have been necessary was a little attention to certain rules of skin care.

Roberta B., a 35-year-old divorcee, was so ashamed of her skin that she wore heavy make-up along with slacks and long sleeves and refused to bare her skin at the local beaches. When she carried out a simple program utilizing some of the principles outlined in this chapter, veins and blemishes disappeared and her itchy, splotchy skin was replaced with a glowing, golden skin that was a delight to see and touch. Even her personality and her way of life changed. She became proud rather than ashamed of her body, and she switched to the modern mini fashions. She looked ten years younger than most women her age.

Much unhappiness results from ugly, unhealthy skin. Nothing will break down self-confidence more than "bad skin." This doesn't have to happen to you. With a little knowledge and a little effort, you can keep your skin healthy and youthful in appearance. With "good skin," you can get more out of life, and you can be proud of the way you look.

TOO MUCH SUN CAN AGE YOUR SKIN PREMATURELY

Everyone knows that sunlight builds good health and that a sun-tanned skin is more pleasing to the eye than a milky-white skin that accentuates veins and blemishes. Sunlight even helps to cure a few skin diseases, such as psoriasis and athlete's foot. Few people seem to know, however, that *too much sun can age the skin prematurely.*

A moderate tan is fine. Everyone should expose his skin to the sun often enough to maintain a light tan and to keep the skin thick enough to hide surface veins. But when the skin is baked day after day in order to maintain a dark tan, the skin thickens excessively. Chemical processes are activated which actually *speed* the aging process in the skin. Look at the skin on the back of a farmer's neck, for example, or the face and hands of a fisherman.

Don't stay in the sun any longer than necessary to maintain a light tan. Stay in the shade the rest of the time. A dark tan is simply not worth the price of prematurely old skin and possible skin cancer.

How to Sun Bathe Safely

When you sun bathe for the first time in several months, be careful not to burn your skin. A sunburn is *bad* for your skin, and it can make you ill. Expose your skin to the sun's rays for only a few minutes the first day, and then gradually increase the exposure each day until you have a pleasing, moderate tan.

Some suntan lotions help to prevent sunburn by filtering out some of the burning ultraviolet rays, but don't depend upon them. Time your exposures by the clock so that you won't overexpose your skin. If you begin with short exposures, you can be guided by the effects of the sun in increasing your exposure from day to day.

If you're accustomed to sun bathing in a polluted atmosphere, you will misjudge the intensity of the sun's rays in a non-industrial area where the air is clean and clear. Ultraviolet rays can filter through haze and fog, but not through pollution. For this reason, you should reduce your usual exposure to the sun when you leave the city to sun bathe.

Greasy suntan oils and creams applied over the entire body can interfere with sweating and contribute to heat stroke. So don't sit around all day with cream smeared all over your skin, even if you sit in the shade.

Ultraviolet Lamps Can Be Dangerous

If you'd like to maintain a little tan during the winter, you can use an ultraviolet lamp. You should remember, however, that ultraviolet rays do not give off heat, so there is no sensation to warn you when you have had enough. A burn may not become evident until as long as three or four hours after an overexposure. For this reason, exposures must be carefully controlled and timed. Don't ever expose your eyeballs to ultraviolet rays. Always close your eyes and cover them with moist cotton pads when you're lying under any kind of sun lamp.

A suntan isn't really necessary for good health, so it may not be necessary to expose your entire body to the sun's rays during the winter—except for cosmetic reasons or to aid in correcting a skin disorder.

An infrared lamp gives off only heat rays and does not tan. So be sure not to confuse the two, especially when taking heat treatments to relieve muscle or joint soreness.

CLEANING YOUR SKIN WITH SOAP

Everybody uses soap these days, and it is undoubtedly necessary for thorough cleansing of the skin. Excessive use of soap, however, might be harmful, and there may be occasions when soap should not be used at all. The skin of a child or an old person, for example, does not produce much oil, so less soap would be required for cleaning. When the skin is dry or chapped, oil rather than soap may have to be used.

As a rule, the face is so oily that it can benefit from frequent washing. The rest of the body, however, produces less oil and therefore needs less washing.

The skin is normally acid, and it produces secretions that protect it and keep it soft and pliable. Since most soap is alkaline, too much washing of normal skin can remove skin oils and neutralize acid secretions, thus depriving the skin of its normal protective mantle. This increases susceptibility to infection and frequently leads to skin irritation.

Strong or highly alkaline soaps are often used to wash away grease and grime, especially around the face and hands, but they should be discontinued when the skin begins to show evidence of chapping or cracking.

Be guided by the condition of your skin in determining how often you should bathe with soap. Except in special cases, always select a mild, nearly neutral soap for bathing. When your skin is dry, use less soap and then rub a small amount of olive oil into your skin after bathing. If you have a skin disease, you may have to use a completely neutral soap to avoid any unnecessary irritation.

I personally bathe twice each day (morning and evening) with mildly alkaline soap, with no bad effects.

Since the skin is less oily during the cold weather, persons who have dry skin cannot use much soap during the winter. It may, in fact, be necessary to clean the skin by applying olive oil (or some other vegetable oil) and then scraping it off with a plastic spatula to clean out the pores. The skin may then be rubbed lightly with a moist wash cloth.

Older persons whose skin tends to be dry may have to limit the use of soap to their hands, face, scalp, feet, and groin and then apply a small amount of olive oil to the skin following a fresh-water rinse.

A superfatted soap, which is low in alkali and rich in wool fat, may help replace the oil lost in washing. A little lemon juice in a tub of clean water will help restore the skin's protective acid coating.

KEEPING YOUR NOSE CLEAN

As we grow older, the pores and fat glands around the face and nose sometimes enlarge. If oil is allowed to accumulate in these pores when they have been clogged with dirt, dead skin, or soap, the pores may become even larger, causing huge unsightly blackheads. For this reason, it may be a good idea to clean the pores of your face a couple of times each week by gently pressing out the contents after an evening shower. Dabbing a little alcohol over the empty pores will prevent infection.

CLEANING WITH OATMEAL WATER

When the face and hands are too chapped or irritated to tolerate soap and water, they can be cleaned with oatmeal water. Just boil a small sack of oatmeal in a gallon of water for about five minutes. A handful of oatmeal in a porous cotton bag should be adequate.

Oatmeal water cleans better than plain water, and it leaves a protective film on the skin.

HARD WATER AND YOUR HAIR

Whenever possible you should use soft water when washing, especially when washing your hair. The alkali in soap combines with the magnesium and calcium salts in hard water to form an insoluble soap that clings to the scalp and the hair. This makes the hair dull, stiff, and difficult to manage.

Rain water is soft water, but few people would go to the trouble of collecting enough water to wash and rinse their hair.

If you don't have soft water in your home, you can use an acid rinse to remove the hard soap. The juice of a lemon in a basin of water, or one teaspoonful of white vinegar to each glass of water poured into a basin, followed by a fresh-water rinse, will wash away hard salts and minerals. This will leave the hair soft, lustrous, and easy to manage.

Some modern, synthetic detergents are completely neutral and will not combine with hard-water salts, but I usually recommend plain, mild soap and soft water. There's always a possibility of an allergic reaction to a chemical detergent.

HOW TO ELIMINATE ACNE, BLACKHEADS, PIMPLES, AND BLEMISHES

If your face is plagued by blackheads or acne, chances are your skin is excessively oily. Acne in teenagers, for example, is usually triggered by hormones that cause excessive production of a thick oil that clogs oil glands and pores. Some adults who have only moderately oily skin sometimes develop acne-like eruptions. The oil simply hardens to form plugs that prevent the oil glands from draining. If skin grows over a clogged pore, a whitehead may form. If the outer portion of the plug is exposed to air, the oil combines with oxygen to form a blackhead. In either case, if oil production is excessive, the trapped oil forms red, swollen bumps.

Frequent washing with a moderately alkaline soap is necessary to keep the oil in the pores dissolved. The face should, in fact, be washed as many times as necessary to keep the skin dry.

Applying hot, moist towels to the face will soften oil plugs so that they can be pressed from the pores. Such cleansing should be done at night, following a warm soap-and-water shower. This will remove most of the bacteria on the skin, thus reducing the chances of infection. And if done just before bedtime, you won't have to go out in public with a splotchy, red face. Always dab your face with alcohol after cleaning out the pores.

Creams and oils should never be used to clean an oily, acne-ridden face. Pressing more oil into the pores will simply aggravate the clogged skin. Just stick to plain soap and water—and bathe your face as often as you can.

Bathe under a shower rather than in a tub whenever possible. A flow of water from your head to your feet will wash germs, dirt, oil, and dead skin down the drain for a better bath and a cleaner skin.

Let Your Skin Breathe

Pancake make-up should never be used on the face, expecially when it is spotted by eruptions. The skin must *breathe* to be healthy, and the pores must be left open to secrete oil and to eliminate toxins.

I've seen many adult women who were suffering from acne-like eruptions around their chin and cheeks because of constant use of smothering make-up.

The skin of the face looks much better if it is lightly tanned and free of heavy make-up.

Other Causes of "Bad Skin"

Constipation can aggravate a skin disorder by forcing the skin to eliminate more than its share of toxins and wastes. So be sure to read Chapter 5 for instructions on how to keep your bowels healthy and active.

Too much sugar in your blood encourages infection. So go easy on sugar and candy. If you remember what you learned in Chapter 3, you know that your sweet tooth should be satisfied by fresh, natural sweets. If you ever develop a persistent skin rash or infection, have your blood sugar checked for possible diabetes.

Eliminate all soft drinks and pastries. Any processed or artificial food can be a potential cause of skin trouble. If you have acne or some type of persistent skin eruption, check your diet for possible allergies. Milk, eggs, wheat, nuts, chocolate, pork, cheese, bananas, tomatoes, onions, citrus fruits, and shell fish sometimes cause trouble. If you suspect that any of them are causing an allergic rash, eliminate them from your diet for a while and see what happens.

Artificial cosmetics and lotions can also result in an allergic skin reaction. Use them as little as possible. Eliminate them altogether when you're having skin trouble.

Iodized salt, cough medicines containing iodides, and headache remedies or sedatives containing *bromides* can aggravate acne.

If you suffer from acne, it's all right to empty some of the clogged pores by pressing them gently after bathing the skin. But *don't ever squeeze a swollen "bump."* If an infection is forced deeper into the tissues, a boil or carbuncle might develop. A physician can drain deep acne bumps with a special instrument without spreading the infection.

HOME CARE FOR HOUSEWIFE'S ECZEMA

About 15 percent of all people complaining of skin trouble have housewife's eczema, or itching, redness, and crusty formations on the skin around the hands and fingers. No one knows for sure what causes this disease, but if the hands are protected from exposure to dish water, detergents, metal polishes, floor waxes, furniture polishes, house dust, vegetable and fruit juices, and other possibly irritating substances, the skin will usually heal in a week or two.

The hands can be protected by wearing cotton-lined rubber gloves when washing dishes, and loose-fitting cotton gloves for other chores. It's not a good idea to keep the hands covered for more than 15 or 20 minutes at a time, however, since accumulation of perspiration might aggravate the raw skin. Remember that skin must breathe to eliminate wastes and toxins. Creams and greases should be avoided whenever possible.

Itching can be relieved by immersing the hands in cold water for a minute or two and then letting them dry by evaporation.

Dipping the hands in cold water that contains corn starch may help relieve severe itching. When the skin is excessively dry, a tablespoonful of vegetable oil in a pan of cold water will "oil" the skin. In either case, the hands should be allowed to dry by evaporation.

HOW TO RELIEVE ATHLETE'S FOOT

Athlete's foot, in which the skin around the toes and the bottom of the foot is red, itchy, or blistered, is caused by a fungus. Just about everybody harbors this fungus. It's everywhere. No matter how often you wash your feet, you won't be able to get rid of the fungus entirely.

Not everyone is susceptible to athlete's foot. But those who do develop the disease will experience a recurrence just about every time they bottle up their feet in shoes and socks that allow perspiration to accumulate around the toes.

The fungus that causes athlete's foot thrives on wet, soggy skin. Once it gets started, it literally eats the skin from between the toes. The only way to stop the infection is to keep the feet dry and well ventilated. This means that in the summer you should wear perforated shoes or sandals with thick, white cotton socks that will absorb moisture. Expose your feet to sun and air as often as possible.

Always dry your feet, expecially between the toes, as thoroughly as you can after bathing. Sprinkle your toes and feet with medicated foot powder before putting on your shoes and socks or before going to bed. If the infection keeps recurring, you may have to insert lamb's wool between your toes to keep them dry.

If you can manage to keep your feet dry at all times, you can control or prevent the growth of fungus. If the infection becomes worse in spite of all you do, your doctor can prescribe special medication.

The skin on your feet is just as important as the skin on your face. If you allow fungus to feed on your feet, cracked skin and secondary infection can cripple you just as surely as stepping on a rusty nail. You can prevent all of this by making sure that you don't walk around with sweat-soaked feet.

A SIMPLE TREATMENT FOR CORNS

A corn is simply a build-up of the outer, horny layer of the skin. Most corns occur when bad foot posture or improperly fitted shoes constantly irritate the skin over a bony portion of the foot. The skin simply thickens in order to build a protective pad. If the irritation is removed, the corns will disappear. So the first thing you have to do is to make sure that your shoes are properly fitted and that you maintain good foot posture (see Chapter 13).

Hard corns can be softened by soaking them in hot, soapy water. They may then be trimmed or filed—if care is taken not to expose sensitive flesh.

Certain chemical corn removers, such as salicylic acid in

collodion, can be used if they do not soften or macerate the skin around the corn.

If you are a diabetic, you should not attempt to use home treatment on any foot condition that might become infected. A chiropodist or podiatrist can remove painful corns safely.

A WORD ABOUT DEODORANTS

The apocrine sweat glands under the arms and in the genital area produce perspiration that contains a great deal of organic matter. When perspiration in these areas is not exposed to circulating air so that it can evaporate, the bacteria normally found on the body feed on the organic matter and produce body odors.

For the most part, the apocrine glands are active only as long as the sexual glands are active. This means that the older you become the less body odor you have, even with less bathing. Of course, there are many elderly couples who remain sexually active far into their eighties and nineties. If you should be so fortunate, a daily bath won't prove to be any inconvenience at all.

There are other types of sweat glands in the groin area and under the arms that necessitate occasional bathing, but they do not cause as much odor as the sexually-associated apocrine glands.

Since most of us dress and work in such a way that little or no air circulates under our arms, it's usually necessary to use a deodorant to prevent offensive odors. It should be used only under the arms, never over large skin surfaces. Remember that perspiration is essential in maintaining a normal body temperature and in eliminating waste. *Don't try to substitute deodorants for soap and water.*

HOW TO DRESS SENSIBLY

Try to wear clothing that won't shut off the flow of air to

your skin. Tightly woven, close-fitting garments that cover the entire body can literally suffocate your skin. Be sensible. Be guided by comfort rather than by the prevailing fashion. Leather pants or a leather blouse, for example, should be strictly forbidden. I once saw a popular rock-and-roll singer give a performance in a leather suit. Perspiration poured from his face, and the heat from the television lights nearly baked him alive. Don't ever be guilty of using such poor judgment.

Trousers so tight that they squeeze the hips together are frequently a cause of foul-smelling and itching fungus or bacterial infection in the crevices between the buttocks and the thighs. Lack of air and bottling up of perspiration literally cultivate the type of fungus that causes "jockey itch" or "athlete's bottom." Yet, it is the style among men to wear close-fitting trousers with narrow cuffs. I personally prefer trousers with pleats, so that when I sit down the trousers won't clamp around my hips and squeeze my flesh.

The maxiskirts now being peddled to our women are an insult to human intelligence. In addition to creating a hazard from possible entanglement or fire, they shut out sunlight and air.

During the summer, try to wear loose-fitting cotton clothing. Expose as much of your skin as possible to light and circulating air. Your whole body will benefit, and your skin won't be blemished, soggy, or offensive to the eye or the nose.

DANDRUFF CAN BE CONTROLLED

Everybody has a little dandruff, since the scalp, like skin in other portions of the body, is continuously shedding bits of dead tissue. These bits of skin would hardly be noticed if they didn't combine with scalp oil and dust. Since the scalp is the oilest portion of the body, it must be washed at least twice a week to prevent a visible build-up of dandruff.

When dandruff is unusually heavy or severe, more frequent

washing is necessary. You should, in fact, wash your hair as often as necessary to remove all dirt, dandruff, and excess scalp oil. Olive oil mixed with glycerin may be used to soften fatty accumulations on the scalp before washing. Just rub it in and let it soak for a while before applying soap and water. In some cases, it may be necessary to soap and rinse the scalp several times during a bath in order to remove caked oil and dandruff. A highly alkaline soap may be more effective than a mild soap.

I doubt that it would be possible to wash the scalp too much, since it is constantly secreting oil. But if you think your hair is too dry, you can moisten it with a little olive oil and glycerin.

Brushing your hair frequently with a soft brush will keep dirt-catching oil and dandruff from accumulating on the scalp.

Dandruff may occasionally be caused by psoriasis or some other skin disorder, so it might be a good idea to see a dermatologist when severe dandruff is accompanied by itching or crust formation.

Don't worry about becoming bald if you have dandruff. One has nothing to do with the other.

KEEP YOUR NAILS ATTRACTIVE

Nutrition is important in keeping your nails healthy and attractive. Dry and brittle nails, for example, may result from a deficiency in Vitamin A, calcium, protein, or thyroid hormones.

Occasionally, an allergic reaction to nail polishes or cleaners may result in disease of the nails. It's not at all uncommon for fungus or ringworm to infect the nails and cause thickening or deformity.

For the most part, the appearance of your nails depends upon how well you care for them physically. If you bite your nails, for example, they'll look terrible, no matter how well nourished you are.

The cuticle should be pushed back frequently so that it will not be pulled forward as the nail grows. A dull instrument should be used to clean dirt from under the fingernails. If you scrape the under side of the nail with a sharp instrument, the tiny scratches will collect dirt that will be difficult to remove.

If you have dry hands, avoid prolonged exposure to soapy water, especially dish water. Apply a little olive oil, or some other vegetable oil, to the base of the nails each day to prevent nail deformity caused by a "dry" nail bed.

Ingrowing toenails are usually caused by improper nail trimming or tight shoes. A chiropodist can cut out the ingrown portion of the nail and then use a special packing to prevent regrowth. The nail of the big toe should be cut fairly straight across so that the corners of the nail won't grow out into the flesh.

SUMMARY

1. If your skin is normal, you can keep it clean by bathing regularly with plain soap and water, followed by a cool rinse and a brisk towel rub.

2. An oily face, marred by blackheads or acne-like eruptions, should be washed frequently with alkaline soap and warm water. The skin must be kept dry and the oil in the pores must be dissolved before it hardens.

3. Dry skin should be washed only occasionally (with neutral soap), followed by the application of a small amount of olive oil.

4. Old people and children do not need to use soap as often as the average adult.

5. Persons suffering from inherited dry skin may have to clean their skin with fresh water mixed with a little vegetable oil.

6. A little lemon juice added to a fresh water rinse will help restore the protective acid coating on normal, washed skin.

7. More sun than required to maintain a moderate tan will age the skin prematurely.

8. When you must use hard water to wash your hair, a little lemon juice or white vinegar in a fresh water rinse will remove salts and minerals that stiffen and dull the hair.

9. Athlete's foot is caused by a fungus that feeds on moist, soggy skin. Dry your feet and your toes after every bath and keep them dry by sprinkling them with powder.

10. Since dandruff is usually associated with an oily scalp, frequent washing with a mildly alkaline soap may be necessary to remove oil and dead skin caked on the scalp.

13

How to Help Yourself in Relieving the Symptoms of Aging Chronic Ailments

No matter how long you live or how well you take care of yourself, there are certain common, chronic ailments that you cannot avoid completely. Arthritis, headache, nervous tension, backache, varicose veins, foot trouble, and thinning hair, for example, are commonly associated with the aging process. All of them tend to grow progressively worse if you don't do something about them.

In this chapter, you'll learn how to help yourself to relieve the symptoms of a variety of common ailments. If you would like to have a more detailed guide in the use of self-help techniques for preventing and relieving all sorts of aches and pains, be sure to read my book *A Chiropractor's Treasury of Health Secrets,* published by Parker Publishing Company, West Nyack, New York. In the meantime, I'll reveal several valuable health secrets that you can use *now* to aid your efforts in building youthful health and vigor.

A SIMPLE WAY TO RELIEVE STIFFNESS CAUSED BY ARTHRITIS

There are several types of arthritis, but osteoarthritis is the type most often associated with the aging process. Symptoms usually begin after the age of 40, and often appear first in the hands. Joint stiffness and fleeting pain may be the first indication that something is wrong. The stiffness may be worse in the morning or after prolonged resting.

Osteoarthritis can strike any joint, particularly those that have been injured or subjected to a great amount of wear and tear. A person who performs heavy labor, for example, might develop spinal arthritis. A pianist might develop the disease in his hands. A build-up of calcium in ligaments and around the edges of the joint forms bony spurs and ridges that become a permanent part of the bone. When the hands are affected, bony growths may appear as knots around the finger joints. There is no treatment that will remove these growths. This is one reason why doctors say there is "no cure" for arthritis.

Osteoarthritis rarely cripples, however, and there is a great deal that you can do to relieve symptoms and to prevent the disease from becoming worse.

A Movement a Day Keeps Adhesions Away

You can actually "warm up" a stiff arthritic joint by taking a small amount of exercise. An increased flow of warm blood thins tissue fluids and makes stiff tissues more pliable. The movement combined with the heating effect of the blood can restore normal movement better and faster than any "arthritis medicine" you can buy.

Too much movement or exercise, however, can aggravate an arthritic joint by irritating inflamed joint surfaces. Prolonged unaccustomed activity may, in fact, be damaging. So while you should exercise to relieve stiffness, you should be careful not to do too much. Just try to put the affected joints through a full range of movement several times a day. This will prevent the development of the type of adhesions that cause *permanent* stiffness; that is, the type of stiffness that cannot be relieved by warming up the joints.

How to Apply Moist Heat

Simple moist heat, applied with towels that have been wrung out in hot water, will usually relieve the symptoms of osteoarthritis. In fact, moist heat may be more effective than most of the electronic treatments offered in a doctor's office. Best of all, it can be applied safely at home by anyone.

A 76-year-old woman who complained of back pain, stiffness, and muscle spasm caused by arthritis found that moist heat applications applied each morning before she got out of bed would relieve her symptoms for the rest of the day. It may do the same for you if you have chronic, "incurable" osteoarthritis.

Dry heat is not nearly as effective as moist heat, so don't try to get by with only a heating pad. Dry heat is dissipated by the circulation of blood just beneath the skin, but when heat is combined with moisture, a reflex effect through nerve fibers dilates blood vessels deep within the tissues.

If you have arthritis in your hands, you may simply immerse them in hot water. Other joints may be wrapped or draped with hot, moist towels. For large surfaces such as the back, the towels can be kept hot by covering them with an insulated heating pad or by heating them with the rays of an infrared bulb or lamp. (See Figure 13-1.)

When you do use moist heat, try to apply it for about half an hour two or three times a day. Flannel, which is made from a combination of cotton and wool, is best for holding both heat and moisture.

QUICK RELIEF FOR HEADACHES

One of the biggest causes of premature aging today is nervous stress and strain, which is also a common cause of headache.

No matter what your age might be, a build-up of tension may occasionally tighten the muscles on the back of your

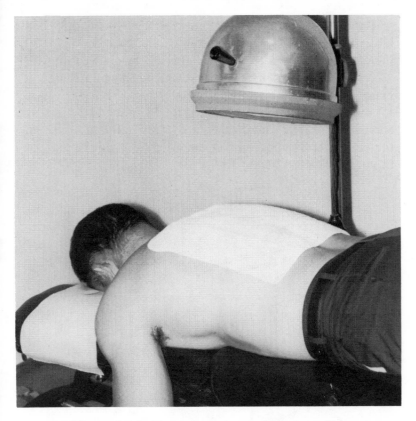

Figure 13-1 *Moist heat is much more effec-tive than dry heat in relieving the symptoms of arthritis.*

neck enough to cause a tension headache. When this happens, there is a simple treatment that you can use at home or at work that will usually relieve your symptoms.

Try a Little Neck Traction

If you suffer from chronic headaches that are not caused by organic disease, you should try a little neck traction. Probably about 95 percent of all headaches are caused by tension, and most of these are triggered by prolonged contraction of the muscles on the back of the neck.

Tight and inflamed neck muscles can be relaxed and loosened by placing a light stretch on the neck for 15 or 20 minutes once or twice each day. This can be done easily with a "cervical traction" head harness, which can be purchased in many drug stores or a surgical supply store. You won't have to use very much weight. Ten to 15 pounds is usually enough. You simply fasten the harness around your head, run the cord over a pulley, and let the weight pull on the muscles of your neck. (See Figure 13-2.)

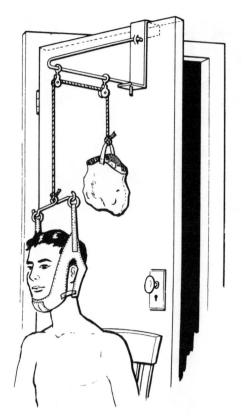

Figure 13-2. *Doorway traction can be used anywhere to relieve tension headache.*

If you want to apply the traction in your office or at work, you can use doorway traction in a sitting position. If you use traction at home, you may prefer to use bed traction so that you can lie down and rest.

If you don't have regular traction equipment, a member of the family can stretch your neck for you. Just lie on your back across a bed and let someone pull on your head. The person applying the traction should cup his hands around the base of your skull and pull very slowly until your neck is stretched as far as it will go (without dragging you across the mattress). A gentle pull should be maintained for several seconds and then slowly released. The pull may be repeated several times in succession.

A fifth-grade school teacher who developed a tension headache "just about every day" found that a few minutes of neck traction in the cloak room would abort the headache by relaxing the muscles of his neck. "If I can prevent those headaches," he said, "I can prevent those nervous rigors I sometimes have when the kids get a little wild."

Traction on your neck should never be painful. It should, in fact, be comfortable and relaxing. One application of traction might relieve an acute headache. If you suffer from recurring headache, however, you should probably submit to traction each day for at least two weeks.

RELAX YOUR MUSCLES TO RELAX YOUR NERVES

Everybody suffers from occasional nervous tension. There are some people who are constantly nervous and tense. Nothing is more damaging to health than unrelieved nervous tension. Organs break down and the aging process is accelerated. Death may occur from a heart attack or from the failure of an important organ. "Nerves" drain energy and vitality from the body.

Fortunately, there is a simple way to relax your nerves by relaxing your muscles. If you can learn to break your tension each time it builds, you can *prevent* illness and aches and pains caused by inflamed nerves and muscles.

Technique for Relaxing Muscles

Several times each day, or when you begin to feel tight and tense, you should let your muscles sag lifelessly. Let your whole body become as limp as a rag. It's important to make sure that *all* of your muscles are relaxed, even the muscles of your face. If you can master the art of complete relaxation, you'll be able to quell the nervous storm that tends to build throughout the day, and your organs will be relieved of damaging stress.

I've known many people who could relieve abdominal pain, upset stomach, headache, muscle spasm, neuritis, hives, and other symptoms simply by relaxing their muscles. Even if you don't have any complaints, you should lie down on the floor occasionally and practice relaxing your muscles until you're satisfied that you can relax on a moment's notice.

A SPECIAL POSTURE TO RELIEVE BACKACHE

If you suffer from chronic backache, you should read my book *Backache: Home Treatment and Prevention* (published by Parker Publishing Company, West Nyack, New York) for all the details of a comprehensive self-help program. In the meantime, there is a simple, restful posture that you can assume that will usually relieve the pain and pressure of postural-type backache.

Sofa Traction

Lie down on the floor and drape your legs over the arm of a sofa (or chair). Scoot up close to the end of the sofa so that your thighs will be nearly vertical while the sofa arm is supporting the back of your bent knees. This posture will reverse the effect that gravity has on the muscles and joints of your back, and it will relieve the pull of hip flexors on your lower spine. (See Figure 13-3.)

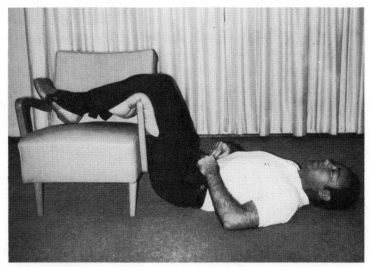

Figure 13-3. *Draping your legs over the arm of a sofa will relax muscles and relieve pressure on joints and nerves in your lower spine.*

You can get a little additional traction on your spine—and relieve pressure on nerves—by placing a pillow between your knees and the sofa arm so that your hips will be lifted an inch or two off the floor. Just lie relaxed in that position for about ten minutes.

I have many patients who use the sofa posture to relieve leg pain as well as backache. An accountant who suffers from a degenerated disc, for example, keeps nerve and joint pain relieved by using sofa traction two or three times a day—right in his office. The next time you have a backache from being on your feet all day, drape your legs over the arm of a sofa and see if you don't get some immediate relief.

HOW TO DRAIN VARICOSE VEINS

Most people who have varicose veins are born with "bad

veins" that have weak valves. Ordinarily, the valves in the veins allow blood to flow in one direction only—that is, toward the heart. When a valve fails, especially in the legs, blood backs up in the veins in response to the pull of gravity. This causes the veins to become large and swollen with blood—a ghastly look of old age.

In some cases, varicose veins cannot be prevented, but there is a great deal that you can do to relieve the pressure in the enlarged veins and recapture your look of youth.

Elevate Your Legs

The easiest and most obvious thing to do to drain the blood out of varicose veins is to elevate your legs. All you have to do is lie down and prop your feet up on a chair so that your legs are higher than your abdomen—and the more often you do this the better. (See Figure 13-4.)

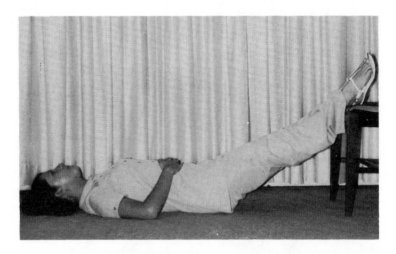

Figure 13-4. *Elevating the legs will drain stagnant blood out of swollen varicose veins.*

If you are a woman, you can wear elastic "support hose" that will keep the veins compressed so that they won't swell with blood. A man who has a bad case of varicose veins can wrap his legs with elastic bandages after elevating his legs.

Regular exercise, such as walking or swimming, will help pump blood through leg veins. The underwater hydrovascular exercises described in Chapter 6 are great for reducing the pressure in leg veins and for stimulating the circulation of blood.

Nothing will mar your youthful appearance more than blue, lumpy varicose veins. You may be able to prevent such disfigurement by doing nothing more than walking and elevating your legs each day.

FIGHTING THE COMMON COLD

Basically, there is no cure for a cold. Once a cold develops, the germs must be destroyed by the body's own defenses. If you are healthy, you will recover from the effects of a cold infection in one or two weeks. If you are run-down or unhealthy, cold symptoms may linger for months, and other types of infections may develop.

Follow all the suggestions outlined in this book for building youthful health and vigor and you will automatically erect a defense against the cold germ. There may be occasions, however, when your resistance to infection will be a little low. And if you are exposed to someone who has a cold during this time, you will probably pick up the infection.

Cold germs are everywhere, but they are not usually strong enough to invade a healthy body. Once they do break through the body's defenses, they become stronger and more virulent by feeding on the body. This is one reason why it's so easy to "catch" someone's cold.

There is something special that you can do to kill cold germs that might be roaming the passageways of your nose and throat. Try it the next time you have even the slightest suspicion that you may have inhaled someone else's cold germs.

The Vinegar-Vapor Treatment

Put a small pot of water on the stove. When the water begins to boil, add just enough vinegar to give the steam vapor a comfortably acid smell. Then inhale the steam off and on for a minute or two. The moisture and the acid fumes will destroy those cold germs that haven't already buried themselves in your throat.

This vinegar-vapor treatment is especially valuable during the winter months when you are forced to breathe hot, dry air in overly heated rooms that are shared by several people.

Eating *garlic* during the "cold season" may also offer some protection against cold germs, since garlic oil is a natural germicide.

DON'T GROW OLD WITH BROKEN-DOWN FEET

The longer you remain in this world, the greater are the chances that you'll have trouble with your feet. Your feet do a tremendous amount of work. In addition to supporting all of your weight, the bony bridges in your feet must function as levers in moving you from one place to another.

Improper use of your feet can strain muscles and tendons and break down the delicate archwork of bones. When this happens, a pair of crippled, "old" feet can create pain and disability that will show as plainly on your face as in your step. Lines of distress may eventually become permanent wrinkles. If you are constantly annoyed by broken-down feet, you'll look and feel 30 years older than you really are.

A Special Foot Posture

Of all the things you can do to help your feet, there is one special posture that can do more for your feet and your disposition than all the pads and powders:

Stand and walk with your toes pointed nearly straight ahead. Lift up the inside portion of your arch so that your weight is supported on the outside edges of the soles of your feet. (See Figure 13-5.)

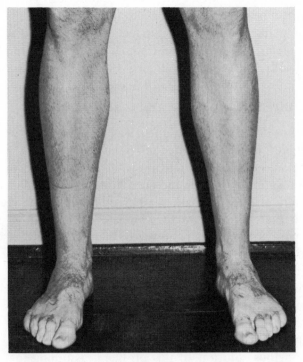

Figure 13-5. *Good foot posture prevents foot trouble and contributes to good body mechanics.*

When you allow your toes to point outward and your feet and ankles to roll inward, the bones and ligaments of the feet are placed under great stress. Also, a rotation transmitted through the legs throws your whole body out of balance, causing backache and other aches and pains—even headache.

A 38-year-old postman who corrected his foot posture reported that chronic knee pains that had defied treatment soon disappeared. "Even my back feels better," he said, "and I haven't had that old muscle spasm under my shoulder blade for several months now."

Make sure that your shoes are properly fitted. Take good care of your feet. Don't let them hold you back in your quest for youthful health and vigor.

If you'd like to exercise your feet, or if you have special foot problems, be sure to read Chapter 10, "How to Improve Your Health with Foot and Leg Care," in my book *A Chiropractor's Treasury of Health Secrets.*

HOW TO ENCOURAGE THE GROWTH OF HAIR

People used to say that baldness was a sign of man's virility. But judging from the increased popularity of hair pieces among men, no man wants to be bald. A thick head of hair makes a man look younger and gives him more confidence.

If you're already "as bald as a billiard ball," there may not be much that you can do to stimulate the growth of new hair. If you still have hair, however, there is something that you can do to prevent the loss of hair and to encourage the growth of new hair.

There are some dermatologists who say that baldness occurs when the scalp becomes so tight that the circulation of blood to the hair roots is restricted. The hair simply falls out from lack of adequate nourishment.

The obvious solution to this problem—assuming that you eat properly—is to stretch and loosen the skin covering the top of your head so that there will be more room for the circulation of blood. Just use your fingertips to move your scalp back and forth and to pinch up the skin. A few minutes of such manipulation each day will be adequate.

Don't wear tightly fitted hats—at least not for long periods of time. Some types of hats fit the head so snugly that they cut off the flow of blood to the hair roots, just as if the head had been encircled with a tourniquet.

SUMMARY

1. There are several common ailments that everyone suffers from at one time or another. All of them can be relieved with home-treatment techniques that will also contribute to the development of youthful health and vigor.

2. The health-building program outlined in all the chapters of this book will *prevent* the development of many types of organic disease.

3. Simple moist heat is very effective in relieving the symptoms of osteoarthritis.

4. Stretching the muscles of the neck will relieve 95 percent of all headaches as well as remove pressure on joints, discs, and nerves.

5. If you can learn to relax your muscles several times a day, you can relieve stress on important organs by preventing a build-up of nervous tension.

6. Lying down and draping your legs over the arm of a sofa will relieve backache, expand discs, and free nerves.

7. You can drain blood out of swollen varicose veins simply by elevating your legs several times a day.

8. Eating garlic or breathing steam vapor spiked with vinegar will kill cold germs in your nose and throat.

9. Protect the bones and ligaments of your feet by walking with your toes pointed straight ahead and your weight supported on the outside edges of the soles of your feet.

10. You can encourage the growth of hair by loosening your scalp with daily fingertip massage.

14

How to Prevent Premature Aging with Restful Sleep

Ronnie D. was a health-conscious engineer who always took his exercise, ate wholesome foods, and followed other health-building rules, such as those outlined in this book. One day, however, he visited my office complaining of fatigue and backache. He hardly looked like the same man he was a few months earlier. His eyes were bloodshot and surrounded by dark circles. His face was thin, pale, and lined, and his blood pressure was high for the first time in his life. I was shocked by his appearance.

"It could be that all I need is a little sleep," he said. "But we have a baby that cries all night, and my wife has been in a mental institution for the last three months. I just haven't been able to get much sleep."

In a few short months, nervous strain and loss of sleep had transformed Ronnie D. from a healthy-looking specimen to a physical wreck.

Few things are as destructive to health as chronic loss of sleep. So no matter what program you might follow to build youthful health and vigor, you'll have to get adequate sleep if you want to succeed.

SLEEP CAN MAKE YOU FEEL WELL AND LOOK YOUNGER

If you want to sleep well every night and then wake up refreshed every morning, you should read this chapter carefully. No matter what type of ailment you might be suffering from, sleep will help you get well. It will also speed your recovery from fatigue and build your defenses against disease.

Only when the body is at complete rest and the mind is relieved of the anxieties that plague us during the day can the body devote its complete attention to its needs. Lack of adequate sleep, in depriving your body of full opportunity to recover from the day's wear and tear, will quickly lower your resistance to infection. Your tissues will age prematurely, and your life span will be shortened. Sleep is just as essential as the food you eat.

WHAT HAPPENS WHEN YOU SLEEP?

Very little is known about sleep. No one really knows what makes us sleep. Physiologists, however, can tell us a little about what happens to the body when we sleep normally. Blood pressure begins to drop, and it reaches its lowest level after about four hours. The pulse rate slows from about 75 to 60. The metabolic rate is greatly reduced. Respiration slows from about 16 breaths per minute to about 12. While everything else slows down, the secretion of sweat increases to aid in the elimination of toxins. The flow of gastric juices increases to speed digestion.

These and many other changes permit the body to heal and cleanse itself, even while it is resting. Energy stores are replenished, and old, wornout tissue cells are replaced by new, youthful cells. The body is literally rejuvenated.

HOW TO GET THE MOST OUT OF YOUR SLEEP

The first four hours of sleep are the deepest. For this

reason, it's very important that your sleep not be interrupted in the hours right after retiring.

Whenever possible, you should sleep at night rather than in the daytime. For some reason not yet clear to medical sleuths, sleep is deeper during night hours. Since most of us have become accustomed to sleeping at night and working during the day, it would be extremely difficult to reverse these habits. Furthermore, unless you have a totally dark bedroom for daytime sleeping, the sunlight filtering through your eyelids would tend to short-circuit the sleep centers in your brain. Noises made by people, machines, and animals would also disturb your sleep. It's difficult to sleep while the rest of the nation is awake.

Persons who work on rotating shifts that require frequent changes from day hours to night hours never really get enough sleep. A paper mill worker on a rotating shift, for example, who suffered from asthma that defied years of medical treatment, was able to cure his trouble by switching to regular daytime working hours. It seems that the inability of his nervous system to adjust to the frequent changes in sleeping hours resulted in a nervous disturbance that constricted the tiny air passages in his lungs.

Conditioning Yourself for Sleep

The ability to sleep soundly for several hours each night must be acquired by conditioning; that is, by going to bed at the same time each night under consistently desirable conditions. Attending late shows, all-night parties, and other functions that bite into the first half of your regular sleeping hours will result in fatigue, loss of sleep, and other symptoms that will disturb your sleep and your sense of well-being for days afterward. This is one reason why some people come back from a vacation more tired than before.

Once you become accustomed to regular sleeping hours,

the simple suggestion of bedtime will be enough to start you yawning and to make your eyelids droop.

How a Housewife Relieved Her Nervous Spells with Sleep

Eugenia D., an overworked housewife and mother with six children, tried unsuccessfully to find a cure for a colon condition and a skin rash she had suffered from for several months. She was also subject to nervous spells that either made her grouchy and hard to live with or blue and depressed. When she began to suffer from insomnia, crying spells, headache, and other symptoms pointing to a nervous breakdown, she hired a housekeeper and made arrangements to supplement a full eight hours of night sleep with a one-hour nap each day after dinner. After only two weeks, her symptoms disappeared and she recovered her emotional stability. The lines in her face disappeared. She looked and felt young again.

How Much Sleep Do You Need to Stay Young and Live a Long Life?

Not all people require the same amount of sleep. For this reason, you cannot be guided entirely by charts that recommend a certain number of sleeping hours for a certain age group. There is some evidence to indicate, however, that *persons who average seven to eight hours of sleep each night have the longest life expectancy.*

People used to believe that the older a person becomes the less sleep he needs. But there is now reason to believe that persons over 60 years of age may need as much as *ten* hours sleep each night, with a one-hour nap in the afternoon.

Some people get along better with a series of naps than with one lengthy night of sleep. Some very busy writers and scientists, for example, find that they are more productive if they sleep only four or five hours at night and then alternately sleep and work during the day. Apparently, the frequent naps are enough to relieve fatigue and refresh the mind and body so that more work can be performed in several daily work periods than in one long working day. I wouldn't recommend such a schedule for the average person, however.

Be guided by the way you feel. If you have regular working hours, you should establish regular sleeping hours and then shorten or lengthen them according to your needs. If you find that you're tired or have difficulty in waking up each morning, for example, and you do not have enough time to catch a few extra winks, try going to bed an hour earlier. If you still do not seem to be getting enough sleep, work your schedule out so that you can take a short nap after dinner.

Persons who have trouble falling asleep at night simply because they aren't sleepy shouldn't sleep during the day. The healthy individual who is getting more sleep than he needs should not expect to sleep at night if he sleeps during the day.

TOO MUCH SLEEP CAN BE BAD FOR YOU

There is now some evidence to indicate that too much sleep may be harmful. Persons who "pass the time" by sleeping, for example, have been found to be more susceptible to certain types of diseases. The mental and physical stupor that results from lying around half asleep all day simply retards the processes of life. You must be *active* to be youthful and vigorous. Get the sleep you need and then get out of bed.

RELAXING YOUR MUSCLES WILL HELP YOU SLEEP

Physiologists now believe that there is a close connection between the nerves and muscles and the sleep centers of the brain. If the muscles are tight and tense, the portion of the brain that produces sleep is not able to function because of the interference of nerve impulses from the muscles. When the muscles relax, however, the tension eases and the mind relaxes. This enables the sleep centers of the brain to function fully and freely so that bedtime will be followed closely by sleep.

If you are a tension-harassed business man, a little exercise at the end of the day will help relieve your tension as well as relax your muscles. Persons who perform labor can relax more completely simply by taking a warm bath before going to bed. Do what you can to avoid going to bed with aching muscles, tense nerves, or an anxious mind.

AVOID STIMULATING DRINKS

There are some people who don't believe that coffee can keep you awake at night. "It's all in your head," they say. "Coffee keeps you awake only if your *think* it will."

Coffee may not disturb everyone's sleep, but it is definitely a nervous system stimulant that can and does keep some people awake. In fact, the caffeine in coffee is such a powerful stimulant that it is sometimes used medically in the treatment of certain nervous and vascular ailments. If you do drink coffee, drink it in the morning so that the effects of the caffeine will wear off before bedtime. Excessive use of coffee can make you so nervous that you'll find it impossible to relax, much less sleep.

Tea is also a nervous system stimulant. It contains a substance called theine that acts very much like caffeine.

A construction foreman who complained about waking up every night around 2 a.m. admitted that he drank "about a gallon" of tea each night. When he quit drinking tea with his evening meal, he was able to sleep soundly all through the night.

Both coffee and tea contain a considerable amount of tannic acid, which may interfere with sleep by retarding digestion and producing constipation.

Cocoa contains theobromine, which is a mild stimulant, along with a small amount of tannic acid. Unlike tea and coffee, cocoa has some food value. Used excessively, however, it may cause indigestion as well as nervousness.

If you drink warm milk at night to soothe an ulcer or to make you sleep, don't flavor it with cocoa. The tannic acid will tend to prevent absorption of the calcium you need to relax your nerves and muscles, and the theobromine may keep you awake.

Cola drinks contain enough caffeine to interfere with sleep. These beverages contain a stimulant taken from the kola nut, which accounts for the instant lift they provide.

If you have trouble sleeping at night, you'd better stick to milk and fruit and vegetable juices for evening beverages. Limit the use of stimulating drinks to breakfast and dinner.

Eating Before Bedtime

A light snack just before going to bed (if you aren't overweight) will aid sleep by diverting blood from your brain to your stomach. Overeating, however, will stimulate the nervous system by overloading the stomach.

A glass of warm milk, in addition to providing nerve-relaxing calcium, tends to relax the entire body by heating and soothing the stomach. A spoonful or two of honey in the milk will add to its sedative effect, and it will act as a mild laxative for the morning toilet.

DON'T TAKE YOUR WORRIES TO BED

When the day's work is done, don't torture yourself by taking your job worries home. Try to erase unsolved problems from your mind. Avoid any kind of mental work that requires heavy concentration after your evening meal. Too much brain work at night will overstimulate your mind and your nerves and make it impossible for you to relax at the flip of a light switch.

When I was a student in college, I found that whenever I studied far into the night I would continue to study in my sleep. Some nervous people review the events of a bad day so intensely that they carry disturbing thoughts right into their dreams.

When the workday is over, think good thoughts. Forget your problems and do the things you like to do. Relax your muscles. When bedtime finally comes, take advantage of the opportunity to place your mind and your body in the peaceful, carefree world of slumberland.

Sleep can give you several wonderful, relaxing, and refreshing hours all to yourself. Don't spoil it by crowding your brain with disturbing thoughts or by worrying about things that are far removed from your bedroom.

GOING TO SLEEP SHOULDN'T BE WORK

Once you've gotten into bed, don't worry about being able to go to sleep. Just relax and enjoy the luxury of being able to rest in the comfort of your own bed. If you'll do this, chances are you'll fall asleep with no trouble at all.

Some people work so hard at *trying* to go to sleep that they prevent sleep by tensing their muscles as well as their minds. Sleep should occur as a natural result of complete relaxation and contentment.

Deep Breathing as a Sleep Aid

Deep breathing exercises while lying in bed may help produce relaxation and sleep. The "blowing off" of carbon dioxide (see Chapter 7) will constrict the blood vessels around your brain to "drug" your mind and body. This will result in a slight dizziness that will tend to make you relax more completely.

Each time you take a deep breath, let your muscles sag when you exhale. Imagine that you're breathing out all your fears, tensions, and anxieties. Let the incoming air flush your brain so that your mind will be as blank as a freshly washed blackboard.

Dress Comfortably

How you dress for bed is important. Wear as little as you can, according to the temperature of your room. I wouldn't recommend sleeping in the nude, however, since this would allow drafts of air to chill skin that might be damp from unabsorbed perspiration.

Select bed clothing that is light and well fitted. It shouldn't be so tight that it "pulls" or so loose that it wraps around you when you turn over in bed.

If the temperature of your room is adjusted to a comfortable 75 degrees or so, you won't need to wear heavy, bulky pajamas or gowns. A light spread or sheet should be adequate for cover.

CONTROLLING THE ENVIRONMENT OF YOUR BEDROOM

Your bedroom should be well ventilated if you want to sleep comfortably and safely. It's impossible to sleep soundly in a room that is hot and stuffy or cold and damp.

Don't let heating or cooling units blow directly onto your bed.

If you have a psychrometer or some other device for measuring the amount of moisture in the air, try to adjust the relative humidity to about 45 percent. When the air is too dry, the membranes in your nose and throat may crack to allow invasion by cold germs. In addition to protecting membranes, an increased amount of moisture in the air tends to weaken the cold virus.

HOW TO COAX YOUR BRAIN TO SLEEP

If you have trouble falling asleep in spite of everything you do to relax your mind and body, take a warm bath, drink a glass of warm milk, and then sit in a comfortable reclining chair with your head back and your eyes closed until you begin to doze. Combining these measures will speed sleep by reducing the flow of blood to your brain.

Make sure that your bed is already prepared for sleeping and that all the nightly chores are completed so that you can go directly from your easy chair to your bed when you begin to get sleepy.

AVOID THE USE OF SLEEPING PILLS

Don't take sleeping pills unless your doctor prescribes them. If you aren't suffering from disease, illness, or injury, you should eventually be able to produce sleep with natural measures. The use of barbiturates and other soporific drugs to make you sleep can be dangerous. The U.S. Public Health Service has reported that more people die from an accidental overdose of sleeping pills than from any other form of drug poisoning. Persons who are drugged or "half asleep" may take an excessive number of pills without even realizing it.

Each night, Americans swallow more than 15 million sleeping pills. Many people become so addicted to these drugs that they cannot sleep without them—and many begin taking pep pills (amphetamines) to stay awake during the day. No one ever died from simple insomnia, but plenty of misguided persons have died from excessive use of "goof balls" and pep pills.

The use of alcohol with drugs is extremely dangerous. Everyone knows that alcohol can give you a hangover, but too few people know that combining alcohol and sleeping pills can *kill* you.

Stay on safe ground and use the natural techniques recommended in this chapter if you want to sleep well tonight, tomorrow, and every night from now on.

SUMMARY

1. Sleep is nature's greatest physician. Nothing will

refresh your mind and body and bolster your defenses against disease like a good night's sleep.

2. The first few hours of sleep are the most important. Make sure your sleep is not disturbed by light, sounds, temperature, and other factors that prevent *deep* sleep.

3. Try to go to bed at the same time each night. If you have trouble getting to sleep, don't sleep during the day.

4. If you can't seem to get enough sleep during regular sleeping hours, in spite of sleeping soundly at night, try taking a nap after dinner.

5. Persons who average eight hours of sleep have the longest life expectancy. Too much sleep, however, can actually contribute to the development of certain diseases.

6. Light exercise helps produce sleep in sedentary persons by producing a mild fatigue and by getting their minds off their troubles.

7. Self-help techniques that relax the muscles also relieve tension so that the sleep centers of the brain can function undisturbed.

8. Don't drink coffee, tea, cocoa, or cola drinks with your evening meal or before bedtime. These beverages contain a nervous system stimulant that might keep you awake.

9. A warm bath and a glass of warm milk at bedtime are effective in producing sleep.

10. If nothing else works, sit up in a slightly reclining chair and read a dull book. This will reduce the flow of blood to your brain and induce sleep by self-hypnosis.

15

A Summary of Basic Rules to Live by
in Maintaining Youthful Health and Vitality

If you follow all of the various programs outlined in the chapters of this book, you'll have all the essential ingredients of an effective youth-building program. There are, however, a few other things that you can do to assure additional protection against disease or injury.

Here are 50 basic rules that you can observe every day of your life. Some of them summarize important points already mentioned in this book. Others cover new but equally important rules of healthful living.

1. A moderate tan will contribute to the beauty of your skin, but remember that too much sun will age your skin prematurely.

2. When retirement days arrive, select a hobby that requires enough physical activity to keep you trim and fit. Recreational exercise is best.

3. Exercising in water is an effective way to tone muscles, reduce body weight, and improve circulation.

4. Eat something raw every day. When you cook vegetables, always put a little aside for use in raw salads.

5. Eat some iron-rich foods every day. Liver, wheat germ, brewer's yeast, whole grain cereals, and the dark-green leaves of vegetables, for example, are rich in iron.

6. If your skin is oily, wash frequently with soap and water. If you have dry skin, however, go easy on the soap and apply a little olive oil to your skin after each bath.

7. Always dry your feet and your groin as thoroughly as possible after each bath and then apply a little powder to absorb perspiration.

8. Wash your hair as often as necessary to prevent a build-up of dandruff.

9. Loosen your scalp daily with fingertip massage to encourage the growth of hair.

10. Use honey, dark brown sugar, or raisins to sweeten foods, beverages, and cereals. Avoid the use of white sugar whenever possible.

11. If you must eat between meals, eat fresh or dried fruits or raw nuts. These foods will provide lasting energy without building up excessive fat stores.

12. Establish regular and convenient toilet hours and stick to them. But never ignore an urge to empty your bowels.

13. Drink several glasses of liquids each day, including water, fruit and vegetable juices, and skim milk.

14. Every meal should include at least one food that's rich in cellulose. This will provide an indigestible residue that will stimulate bowel function.

15. Eat fresh, natural foods whenever possible. Avoid refined, synthetic, or preserved foods. Don't "eat out" every day unless you have to. Select wholesome, properly prepared foods.

16. Reduce the amount of animal fat in your diet to a minimum. Try to eliminate fried and greasy foods altogether. If you do use cooking oil occasionally, use liquid vegetable oil.

17. Eat more chicken and fish. They're just as rich in protein as beef, and they're low in saturated fat.

18. Take some form of exercise regularly—at least twice a week. Endurance exercise that increases respiration and heart rate is best for keeping a lean body and building a strong heart.

19. When lifting a heavy object, always squat down with your back flat and lift with your legs. Keep your spine as upright as possible.

20. When standing and walking, keep your toes pointed nearly straight ahead with your weight supported on the outside edges of the soles of your feet.

21. Always use moist heat rather than dry heat when treating sore muscles or arthritic joints at home.

22. Eat a minimum amount of fat and only a small amount of carbohydrate. Increase your intake of protein foods that aren't prepared with grease or oil. If you're overweight, you can get low-fat protein from skim milk, cottage cheese, lean meat, chicken, and fish.

23. Basically, a balanced reducing diet should be made up of lean meat, fruits, vegetables, green salads, cottage cheese, and skim milk.

24. The most effective formula for a lean, trim body is this: natural food + exercise. Resistive exercise will keep your bones as well as your muscles strong.

25. Don't ever take a deep breath and hold it during an exertion. Always exhale during any effort that requires contraction of the abdominal muscles.

26. Practice your deep breathing exercises *after* you have taken a little exercise. This will prevent dizziness from overbreathing or hyperventilation.

27. If you suffer from overbreathing caused by nervousness or anxiety, breathe into a paper bag occasionally in order to restore the proper balance of carbon dioxide and oxygen in your blood.

28. Make sure that the air where you sleep and work is clean and free of exhaust fumes. Whenever possible, adjust

the relative humidity of your home or office to about 45 percent.

29. Go to an open window several times a day and take a deep breath. This will clean out your lungs, open closed air sacs, and draw venous blood to your heart so that it can be pumped through your lungs for a fresh supply of oxygen.

30. For added insurance in getting all the vitamins and minerals you need, supplement your diet with brewer's yeast, bone meal, desiccated liver, wheat germ, fish liver oil, dried kelp, powdered skim milk, and sun-dried fruits.

31. Make sure that your daily diet includes milk or cheese; meat, poultry, fish, or eggs; fruits and vegetables; and whole grain breads or cereals.

32. When you cook vegetables, use a low flame with as little water as possible for as short a cooking time as possible.

33. Eat a piece of citrus fruit or a tomato every day so that your body will have enough Vitamin C to fight off infection. Remember that this vitamin is easily destroyed by heat, light, air, and other factors, so try to get it from fresh, *raw* fruits and vegetables.

34. Lie down on a slant board several times a day in order to reverse the effect that gravity has on the muscles and joints and the circulation of blood.

35. Remember that walking and other forms of exercise that activate the muscles of the thighs and legs will aid the circulation of blood. Walk as much as you can.

36. Don't overeat. In addition to depriving your brain of the blood it needs to function efficiently, an overloaded stomach places a strain on your heart.

37. Pull your abdomen in as far as you can several times each day. Try to keep your abdomen flat at other times by holding it in a little.

38. Do bent-knee sit-ups or trunk curls at least every other day for protection against hernia and to maintain the tone of the muscles supporting your abdominal organs.

39. Cigarettes and alcoholic beverages can shorten your

life by destroying vitamins and damaging important organs.

40. Always finish a bath or shower by gradually turning down the temperature of the water until it is comfortably cool.

41. The sleep centers of the brain can function better if the muscles are relaxed and the nerves are relieved of tension and anxiety.

42. A warm glass of milk at bedtime induces sleep by diverting blood from the brain to the stomach and by supplying the body with tension-relieving calcium and Vitamin D.

43. Never drink coffee, tea, cocoa, or cola drinks just before bedtime or with your evening meal.

44. Sleep on a mattress that's firm enough to keep your spine from sagging but not so hard that it cannot mold itself to the normal curves of the body.

45. Stretch your spine occasionally by hanging from a chinning bar or a tree limb. You can get a more relaxed form of spinal traction by lying on your back with your legs draped over the arm of a sofa.

46. Never sit for very long in a chair that's so high that the edge of the seat cuts into the back of your thighs.

47. Elevate your legs several times a day in order to drain stagnant venous blood out of distended veins. You can do this effectively by resting your heels up on a wall or on a chair.

48. Make sure that your shoes fit your feet rather than force your feet to fit your shoes.

49. If you're retired and you sit a lot, sit in a rocking chair so that the rhythmical to and fro rocking motion can aid the circulation of blood.

50. Keep this book in your home and read it over and over. If you put into effect what you learn by reading it, you're bound to look better, feel better, and live longer.

How well and how long your body serves you depends almost entirely upon how well you care for it. It's up to you.

Index

A

A, vitamin, to lengthen life, 73-74
A Chiropractor's Treasury of Health Secrets, 208, 220
Abdomen, flat, benefits of for improved blood circulation, 98-101
   sit-ups, importance of, 98-99
   trunk curls, 99-101
Abdominal breathing, 120-121
Acne, how to eliminate, 198-200
Activity as key to weight control, 187-189
Adaptability to earth's environment as determinant of life span, 22
Aging, premature, eating to prevent, 61
Aging process, checking by proper breathing, 118
Ailments, chronic, of aging, relieving symptoms of, 208-221
   arthritis, simple method to relieve, 208-210, 211
   backache, special posture to relieve, 214-215
   cold, common, 217-218
   feet, problems with, 218-220
   hair, encouraging growth of, 220-221
   headaches, 210-213
   nerves, relaxation of, 213-214
   varicose veins, draining, 215-217
Alcohol, danger of for heart, 148-150
Alkalizers and bowel regularity, warning about, 93-94
Alkalizers and vitamin C, 68-69
Amino acids, essential, how to get, 77-78

Anemia, smoking and symptoms of, 132-133
   other causes of, 135-136
Angina pectoris, meaning of, 151
Animal and vegetable fats, balancing in diet, 141-142
Antacids and bowel regularity, warning about, 93-94
Anti-gravity effect of salt-water exercises, 108
Arteries, fat in, as aging to body, 139-140
Arthritis, simple method to relieve, 208-210, 211
Ascorbic acid for beauty and youthfulness, 65-71
Aspirin, excessive use of as interference with blood clotting, 76
Atherosclerosis, meaning of, 139-140
Athlete's foot, 201-202
Autointoxication, 86
Avocation, value of in relieving fatigue, 34

B

B complex, importance of to youthfulness and beauty, 71-73
   drinkers, warning for, 73
   other B vitamins, 72-73
   riboflavin, 72
   "stolen" from body by sugar, 50-51
   thiamine, 71-72
Back treatment, stimulating, 176-177
Backache, special posture to relieve, 214-215

P. 134; Hilda's case

P. 142
P. 144
2 teaspoons of wheat germ oil each day (2 teaspoons each
meal) should supply adequate Vitamin E along with
unsaturated fat. From page 146, 3rd paragraph.
See page 158, too.